DESTINATION FIVE

Robert Lee was Dean of the Faculty of Veterinary Medicine in Dublin's Trinity College for seven years, Inaugural Dean of the School of Veterinary Medicine, University of Zambia, and the Advisor to the Japanese Government's Veterinary Education Project.

A distinguished member of the Royal College of Veterinary Surgeons, (RCVS), and a member of the Veterinary Council of Ireland for fourteen years, Professor Lee has also held positions in Tanzania, the United Kingdom, Nigeria and Zambia. In addition to the fifteen years he spent working on the continent of Africa, he has been involved in many government and academic initiatives concerned with development co-operation overseas. As a member of the Council of the Royal College of Veterinary Surgeons, London, he became Vice-Chairman and, subsequently, Chairman of the RCVS Examinations Committee which is responsible for awarding Fellowships and Diplomas in major specialist areas. He was also a member of the RCVS Panel of Visitors for the inspection and assessment of Veterinary Schools in Great Britain and Ireland.

In Nigeria he was an elected Founder Member of the Nigerian Veterinary Council, the statutory body responsible for the control of the veterinary profession in Nigeria, and President of the Nigerian Veterinary Association. Founder Chairman of the Ireland Tanzania Society, Professor Lee was Technical Consultant to the Irish Department of Foreign Affairs' Smallholders Livestock Development Project on the island of Pemba, Tanzania.

Professor Lee has published widely in scientific journals. His most recent publication has been his contribution to the history of the Veterinary College of Ireland: A Veterinary School to Flourish: The Veterinary College of Ireland 1900-2000 *(ed. W.J.C. Donnelly and M.L. Monaghan; Dublin: Faculty of Veterinary Medicine, 2001).*

DESTINATION FIVE

*Memories of an Irish vet
in wartime Tanganyika*

Robert P Lee

Morrigan

To my daughter Juliet, who encouraged me towards
recording these memories, and to my wife Joyce,
in gratitude for her unfailing support.

first published 2003 by

Morrigan
Killala, County Mayo,
Ireland

© *2003 Robert Lee*

ISBN 0 907677 02 9

Editorial Services by Gillian Brennan
Typeset by Carole Lynch
Printed by Betaprint

A catalogue record for this book is available
from the British Library.

contents

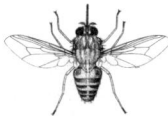

The decorative motif at chapter endings is an illustration of tsetse fly.

foreword

Following a lifetime dedicated to veterinary science and education, Professor Lee has written a fascinating account of the problems confronting those charged with controlling disease in livestock, especially in the developing world. Much of the book deals with disease problems he encountered in Tanganyika in the 1940s; many still prevalent today, such as foot and mouth and African swine fever, are pertinent to current concerns in the European Union.

The real meat of the book covers his experiences as a veterinarian in Tanganyika, firstly at the Headquarters at Mpwapwa where he was in charge of the diagnostic and research laboratories for almost a year and was subsequently responsible for disease control in a province three times the size of Ireland. Written in an easy, self-effacing and often humorous style, one has to marvel at Lee's account of rinderpest vaccine production under primitive conditions and in quantities necessary to immunise thousands of cattle against this virulent viral disease. The biosecurity required to prevent virus used for preparation of the vaccine escaping from the laboratory had the added problem of predators such as lions attacking the donor cattle used for vaccine production!

In Western Province and elsewhere Lee had to deal with diseases such as foot and mouth, trypanosomiasis and East Coast Fever and his descriptions of these are masterful. Nutritional problems exacerbated by drought and the sheer hostility of the environment to the creation of a livestock industry are brilliantly brought out and the reader is left with sensations of the noise, smell and colour of Africa.

This book is compulsory reading for any veterinarian or others with an interest in global animal health problems as well as for nostalgic expatriates and indeed all those interested in Africa.

Professor Sir James Armour, CBE

CHAPTER ONE

Early Days

Family background, and experiences of parents in Ireland's War of Independence. Childhood excursions in north County Dublin when Santry and Finglas were rural villages and Dublin Airport was merely a derelict site of a former British Army flying field. Annual holidays working on relatives' farms in Scotland. Schooldays at St. Andrews College followed by five years at the Veterinary College of Ireland at Ballsbridge.

I was born in Glasnevin on the north side of Dublin during the Irish War of Independence. The first documentary indication I have of my existence is a British Military Permit issued by the Auxiliary Police who were reputedly more sophisticated but even crueller and more treacherous than the notorious Black and Tans. The permit allowed my father, George Angus McLean Lee, to be 'abroad' during the two weeks ending 7 May 1921. Obviously, my father had taken the trouble to obtain the permit from the Castle so that he could fetch our doctor, Dr Winder, if necessary after dark. The Doctor's house was located about half a mile away just outside the Botanic Gardens. In the event, the permit expired the day before I was ready to meet my siblings Angus, Anna and Molly who were respectively two-and-a-half, five and seven years older than me. I remained the youngest member of the family.

My father, who came of solid Scottish farming stock, qualified as a pharmaceutical chemist at the turn of the century whereupon he was offered appointments in both Cork and Jersey. It was fortunate for me that he chose Cork because after a few years there he met Roberta Pearson, a beautiful, tall, black-haired Scottish girl several years younger than himself. She had come from St Andrews to keep house for her brother Andrew. Originally, she was to stay for six months but having met the dapper, energetic pharmacist with a characteristic pep in his step she lingered longer and they were eventually married in 1911. Shortly thereafter, they moved to Dublin where George (or 'Lee' as he was affectionately called by his wide circle of friends, in accordance with the custom of those times) became manager and subsequently the proprietor of Laird's Pillar Pharmacy. The pharmacy was on the corner of Henry Street and O'Connell Street, facing Nelson's Pillar and beside the General Post Office, locating him right next to what would become the focal point for the 1916 Rebellion.

His responsibility at Laird's exposed him to a great deal of violence and pecuniary loss during the War of Independence and the subsequent Civil War. For example, during the War of Independence the British Forces placed an 18-pounder howitzer outside the Pillar Pharmacy and from there bombarded the Gresham Hotel and other buildings on the opposite side of O'Connell Street. The discharge of shells shattered the windows, brought down most of the ceilings and otherwise damaged the structure of Laird's building. During the Civil War the same thing happened again and on both occasions the compensation fell far short of the costs of restoring the building. On one of those occasions, while inspecting the damage inside the building, he was about to be shot as a looter by a drunken Black and Tan and was saved only in the nick of time by a friendly policeman who identified him.

Prior to the Rebellion my parents, as relative newcomers, would not have been particularly sympathetic with the movement for Irish Independence and probably felt that the country should be content to continue to enjoy the material and other benefits of membership of the British Empire. They certainly would have had no sympathy with the philosophy that 'England's adversity is Ireland's opportunity'. However, in common with the vast majority of the Irish people they were shocked by the executions of the leaders of the Easter Rising and the manner in which they were carried out, and with the conduct of the Black and Tans and the Auxiliaries. Consequently, after the establishment of the Irish

Free State my parents were content to stay on and understandably became supporters of Mr Cosgrave's pro-Treaty, pro-Commonwealth Party. Indeed my father greatly admired the excellent work that the Government did in establishing the new State during the twenties. Over the years he often said "There's no doubt, it's a great little country".

As Scots they certainly never regarded themselves as Anglo-Irish or West Britons. However, during our childhood we as members of a small, steadily diminishing Protestant community felt somewhat isolated and not quite full members of the club. Probably one of the most isolating influences was the *Ne Temere* decree that during my childhood required the Protestant partner embarking on a mixed marriage to sign an undertaking to raise any children they might have as Roman Catholics. Consequently, this caused most of the Protestant churches to run dances called 'Socials' exclusively for the young members of their congregations in an effort to decrease the rate at the which the Protestant community was declining. In addition, there were exclusively Protestant or Catholic schools. Despite this level of segregation, my parents and the rest of the family had, of course, the warmest of relations with most of our neighbours and other members of the other persuasion with whom they happened to be brought into close contact.

In 1925, before car-ownership was common, my father bought a brand new, bullet-nosed Morris Cowley tourer and this had a profound effect on our childhood and adolescence during the succeeding thirteen years. He was so attached to it that he could not be persuaded to dispose of it until 1938. During the car's lifetime, it enabled my father and mother to transmit to us their love of the country and their interest in animals. Some of the most enduring memories of my childhood and early teens are the regular expeditions we made to the seaside and the exploration of the countryside in North County Dublin and Meath. In those days, the green fields began just across the Tolka at Glasnevin and the first isolated village was Finglas. To the east it was a country walk from Whitehall to Santry.

On our family's outings to the country my mother enjoyed nothing better than to stop at some wayside cottages to buy really fresh, new-laid eggs which were quite different from the grocers' eggs of those days. These trips were always more frequent during the spring because, long before the advent of intensive poultry farming involving the use of artificial daylight, eggs were in short supply during the winter months. As the days lengthened there was a great flush of egg laying which persisted until the hens became broody. Consequently eggs were dirt-cheap in the spring so that was the season for thrifty housewives with access to the country to preserve new-laid eggs, the fresher the better. They were stored, in our case under the stairs, in great earthenware jars containing a solution of sodium potassium silicate ('waterglass') for use during the winter.

My mother was a great talker and during the course of these visits friendships developed. Before very long my father would become tired of the chat and to my great relief would take Angus and me out 'to stretch our legs'. He was a farmer at heart and as soon as we were out he would set off for the nearest boreen with me in hand in search of cattle while my brother, who even at that early age was a budding fisherman, would inspect the nearest stream for little trout that were seldom there. While it was beef cattle of any breed that my father was looking for, his day was made when he found a herd of Aberdeen Angus. There we would stand on the ditch while he admired the cattle and drew my attention to those with the smallest heads and point out the flatness of their backs, the round hindquarters and the relative shortness of their legs. Plenty of solid meat with little bone! On other occasions, where possible, my brother and I would hunt for tadpoles and newts to take home to our home-made pond in the garden.

In the summer the Morris Cowley enabled all of us to make our annual expedition to Scotland. The preparations were meticulous. Everything had to be oiled and greased, the engine 'decarbonised', carburettor cleaned, dynamo checked and new plugs fitted. Nothing could be left to chance because garages were few and far between. The so-called 'Tryptique' had to be obtained well in advance from Customs with the identification numbers of all the tyres entered thereon to ensure that they would not be replaced with new tyres which were cheaper across the border. The most exciting moment came when the metal carrier that had been hanging in the garage since the previous holidays was bolted onto the back of the car in readiness for the huge hamper that was to carry our belongings, sufficient for an absence of three weeks. The ultimate destination was Strichen in Aberdeenshire but at 25 to 30 mph with a night crossing from Belfast to Ardrossan and stopovers of one or two nights at Mother's relatives in Edinburgh and Tayport it generally took a week to reach our final destination. One of the many high points of the journey was the successful crossing of the Border between Dundalk and Newry after prolonged scrutiny by the authorities on both sides. My brother and I were always excited at the sight of members of the Royal Ulster Constabulary in green uniform with pistols at their belts. The grand finale to the whole journey occurred when we eventually turned off the public road, a mile beyond Strichen, onto the private lane leading up the hill to 'Whitestripe', the farm of my father's eldest brother John. The welcome was always beyond measure but in the early days Angus and I and our youngest cousin, Melita, usually charged out to the steading as soon as we could to see the horses and other animals, including the poultry, to chase rabbits and to play in the hayshed.

When we were older, my sisters and Angus and I stayed at another farm, Tyrie Mains, where there was more accommodation. It was the home of Uncle John Bell, Aunt Nellie and enough cousins to allow each of the Lees to pair off with a Bell of their own age. It was a large farm with its own cotter houses (cottages) for its many farm labourers, at least twelve pairs of horses, its own blacksmith, a carpenter, a steam engine and a mill. The latter served the surrounding farms as did a massive Clydesdale stallion. Mares from nearby farms came to Tyrie for service and from time to time the stallion disappeared with his attendant for days on end to cover mares much further afield. We had the freedom to take the pony and trap to a beach at Aberdour or anywhere else we liked and we occasionally encountered the stallion and his attendant on the road far from home. It was an impressive sight. On their arrival, the Lee cousins were immediately absorbed with great affection into this vibrant community yet we were never allowed to forget that we, as 'townies' with Irish accents, were different. For our part we took great pleasure in reminding them that they were hopeless mimics, whereas we were masters of the doric.

Another person who had a profound influence on my future life was my Uncle Andrew who moved from Cork to Dublin in 1920 to take up a post with the Board of Works. In this post he was, amongst other things, virtually in charge of the Phoenix Park. He and my aunt and my cousin Nancy lived there in Fort Lodge a little to the west of the Magazine Fort. My early memories of him are of a cheery, rotund gentleman full of fun.

Apart from the fact that he was our only uncle in Ireland he was greatly loved by us all, including my mother and indeed my father. I can still see him amply filling my father's large armchair, with his gold watch chain stretched across his ample stomach, while the 'young fry', as he called us, struggled with each other to get a place upon his knees. Once up, the squabbling ceased abruptly as we settled down and listened with rapt attention to wonderful stories of his encounters with tigers in India, and lions and jackals in Africa; all told with an outrageous amount of poetic licence.

His duties in the Phoenix Park endowed him with a key to a private door into the Zoological Gardens and as children we were very privileged to be escorted by him through the Gardens. The keepers held him in high regard and went out of their way to take us behind the scenes to see some of the newborn animals, including cubs of the then world-famous lions of the Dublin Zoo. There is a photograph in a family album of me, aged about three, and a baby chimpanzee, both of us in the arms of a keeper. The principal distinguishing feature is my blonde hair! During my teens I was frequently drawn back to the Zoo where the heat of the lion house and the sight and smell of the caged animals inexorably increased my interest in the tropics. My uncle's wider duties in the Board of Works involved him in the development of other now famous parks throughout the State for which he was for many years remembered. Perhaps one of his most notable contributions was the work he did for the Roman Catholic hierarchy in connection with the preparation of the facilities in the Phoenix Park for the Eucharistic Congress, which was held in 1932. His contribution was graciously recognised by the award of a commemorative gold medal.

During the thirties the economy of the Free State was crippled by the 'Economic War' which broke out following Mr de Valera's refusal to pay the annuities to the British Government. Essentially, these represented the rents that were paid to absentee landlords prior to Independence. The crisis lasted from 1932 to 1938 coinciding with the Great Depression. Throughout this period the cashflow at Laird's was tight and, in common with most of our family friends, we all had to draw in our belts to a very considerable extent. Nevertheless, my parents were still in a position to send the four of us to almost any of the good secondary schools in Dublin.

In September 1933 I moved from our local National School to St. Andrew's College on St. Stephen's Green, on the south side of the city. I was a day-boy and travelled there on the number fourteen tram through the quiet streets of Dublin. A year later I was joined by Angus who, due to asthma, had been advised by doctors to start his secondary education in Edinburgh.

By 1933 St. Andrew's had seen better days. Prior to the foundation of the Irish Free State, the number of students attending had enabled it to win the coveted Leinster Rugby Cup on more than one occasion. The long list of past pupils on the nine panels of the Roll of Honour in the Assembly Hall, honouring those who had served in the First World War, reflected the level to which numbers had fallen. During my time there the student population was about 140. Discipline was poor and staff members in general were not particularly inspiring. However, there were a few exceptional teachers who encouraged us all to live up to the good traditions of the school. The students responded to their enthusiasm and as a result the majority participated actively in sports. Angus and I concentrated mainly on rugby and boxing and were both picked for the Senior Rugby Team which competed respectably against even the largest rugby playing schools for the Leinster Cup, though St. Andrew's had little, if any, prospect of winning.

Boxing was a different matter because our sole purpose was to beat a sworn rival, the team of the Dublin High School, and to win the Ellerker Cup every year. Surprisingly, the Cup had been donated by a Dublin general practitioner, Dr Ellerker, for competition between the two schools. Apparently, in those days, he as a medical man had no scruples about encouraging little schoolboys to spend the winter months preparing themselves for the infliction of physical injury on their peers. The big event was held in a full-sized professional boxing ring in Trinity College, and was attended by large numbers of boys from the two schools. In retrospect, I believe that school boxing has advantages for youngsters that justify the risk of their inflicting physical injury on each other. A boxing ring is a very lonely place for a youngster, especially when he is surrounded by a large audience of his peers. He is completely on his own and it is entirely up to him to get himself out of any predicament that may arise.

7

As mentioned above, discipline was lax to the extent that the school was rather like a club. Only a few of the teachers pressed you to work but if you did not wish to do so that was fine. Such a state of affairs made the first year in university easier for St. Andrew's boys, whereas others who had graduated from more disciplined schools found it harder initially to adjust to the freedom of university life.

Just before I left St. Andrew's I had turned seventeen and in those days one merely had to present a birth certificate to the Local Authority to obtain a driver's licence. Driving tests were unheard of and insurance for young drivers did not seem to be a problem either. By then the Morris Cowley was thirteen years old and, despite the wide horizons and happy memories that it had brought to our childhood, my brother and I were positively ashamed of the old crock whose touring speed was only 25 mph. Nevertheless we appreciated being allowed to borrow it whenever necessary. On one occasion we wound her up to her maximum speed of 35 mph along the straight in the Phoenix Park. I well remember how exhilarated we, and our friends in the back, were by the noise she created at that speed and by the difficulty we had in keeping her on the road. Such jaunts were, of course, unknown to our father.

In the summer of that year my brother who had just completed his first year as a medical student had a serious talk with me in the quiet of our sitting room. By then I had been accepted for admission to the Veterinary College. He thought I had made a mistake and felt that I should try to switch to medicine. He pictured us going into partnership together. We were so close to each other that it was very tempting but by then I had made up my mind. The interest my parents had taken in animals and the course of my life up to then had made my decision irreversible: I was going to be a vet. Moreover, because of the impression my Uncle Andrew's stories had made on me, I would probably end up in the tropics.

That autumn I was admitted to the Veterinary College of Ireland at Ballsbridge to begin the five-year course for Membership of the Royal College of Veterinary Surgeons, London. There was little if any competition for places in those days and the entrance requirements were by no means difficult. The tuition fees of £25 per annum were negligible in comparison with today's, whereas my brother's fee for the Medical School in Trinity College Dublin was almost twice that amount. This state of affairs was a welcome relief to my parents and, indeed, to us all as money was still very tight.

On the first day of term I reported at the given time to the College of Science on Merrion Street where my classmates and I were instructed to wait outside. We did so sitting for almost the rest of the morning in warm sunshine on the broad flight of steps leading into the spacious Entrance Hall of the building that is now the elegantly appointed Government Buildings. The veterinary students were a diverse lot in terms of accents, appearances and personalities, drawn as we were from the four corners of the thirty-two counties and from further afield. A group of Kerrymen, as an example of one extreme, tended to sit together looking suspiciously at the city slickers from Dublin who, in turn, kept their distance from the 'quare fellows' with the Northern accents. Traditionally, some forty percent of the intake came from Northern Ireland and for the majority of them this was probably the first time that members of the two communities there, Loyalists and Nationalists, had met and been given the opportunity to begin to understand each other. Long before the end of their five years at the Veterinary College the differences that had existed between the various strands north and south of the Border became of little significance. After five years of trials, tribulations and much laughter they emerged with one powerful bond in common; they were vets. The unity that this bond gave to the profession in Ireland probably exemplified more fully the Royal College of Veterinary Surgeons' motto *Vis Unita Fortior* than obtained on the other side of the Irish Sea.

During our first year we received our instruction in chemistry, physics and biology at the College of Science and on one afternoon a week we went to the attractive buildings of the Veterinary College at Ballsbridge for animal management. After passing through the impressive arch bearing the legend 'Royal Veterinary College of Ireland' surmounted by a coat of arms displaying the lion and the unicorn, the first building to the left after the caretaker's lodge in those days was the museum. Through the windows, the sight of skeletons of the horse, ox, pig and, best of all, the skull of an elephant complete with tusks, was an exciting reminder that we were to begin real veterinary studies the following year after the somewhat dreary, basic sciences that most of us had been exposed to at school.

The young lecturer in animal management, Des O'Connor, was a gentleman in the best sense of the word and as such was an excellent representative of the other members of the academic staff. At that time they were all civil servants employed by the Department of Agriculture. By virtue of that alone they probably did not enjoy much, if any, academic freedom with which to innovate in such matters as fund raising for the employment of graduate students and the conduct of their own research. Furthermore, the curriculum was set by the Royal College of Veterinary Surgeons so there must have been little opportunity for the teachers to introduce imaginative changes. Nevertheless, they were a competent, dedicated staff and any frustrations they may have had never came through to the students. The efforts they made to impress upon us the importance of maintaining the highest ethical standards within the profession was also impressive.

The students, of course, were a lively lot and only marginally less wild than their counterparts in the three Dublin medical schools. Endless anecdotes, many of them hilarious, could be told but my story here is about Tanganyika, not student life.

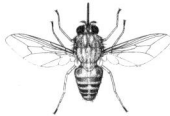

CHAPTER TWO

Recruitment

The author's decision to join the British Colonial Service is copper-fastened during the final veterinary examinations. Bureaucratic and physical difficulties associated with travel between neutral Ireland and wartime Britain. Colourful interviews with the Colonial Office's Recruitment Panel in London during a sub-tropical heatwave.

When the Second World War broke out in 1939 I was about to enter my second year of studies at the Veterinary College. Having been educated at St. Andrew's College, where the teaching had reflected a dual loyalty to both the Irish Free State, as it was then called, and the British Commonwealth, a few of my former classmates soon volunteered for service with the British Forces, even though Ireland had by then declared its neutrality. I continued my studies during the first year of the 'phoney war' while the Nazis and the Allied forces merely faced each other across the Maginot Line, so by the time the real fighting began I was almost into my third year with two to go. By then British veterinary surgeons and students were exempt from military service so, rightly or wrongly, I decided to finish my training.

Eventually, the scheduled day and hour in July 1943 arrived for the final examinations and at precisely 10 a.m. the sealed envelopes containing the first paper were opened simultaneously in Dublin, Liverpool, Glasgow, Edinburgh and London. In due course, the examiners from the Royal College arrived in Dublin at the end of their circuit around the five Veterinary Colleges to conduct the practical and oral examinations.

Having spent the previous summer in Aberdeenshire, as part of a six-month statutory period gaining hands-on experience in farm animal practice, I could appreciate how trying their weary wartime circuit must have been. It involved crossing the Irish Sea in the overcrowded Mail Boat at a slow pace imposed by the overhanging barrage balloon which was intended to give some protection against the possible risk of attack by German dive bombers. On arrival back at Holyhead, which in those days was teeming with warships of various shapes and sizes, they had to endure further rail travel back to London usually with standing room only in compartments and corridors packed to capacity with soldiers, sailors, airmen and civilians who sat for hours on end on their heavy packs or suitcases if they were fortunate enough to have one. Train travel by night was even more tedious. The blackout blinds were tightly drawn and if one dared to pull an edge aside it was pitch dark outside, even when passing through built-up areas, because of the strict observance of the regulations.

Nevertheless, the examiners probably considered their journey to Dublin well worthwhile because even by 1943 Ireland was still, to some extent, a land flowing with milk and honey. We enjoyed abundant supplies of steaks, cream, butter, bacon and eggs to compensate for the almost complete absence of tea, white bread, coal for domestic heating and for the railways with a mere 8 gallons of petrol per month available only to priests, doctors, veterinary surgeons and hackney cars, more or less in that order of priority in the minds of the populace of the time. What a joy it was for visitors from the hungry side of the Irish Sea to sit down to a traditional Irish breakfast instead of tea and toast with a thin smear of butter from their precious ration of an ounce or two per week!

After a satisfying breakfast the examiners were full of bonhomie and they calmed each student with a reassuring smile as he was ushered in to his oral exam. My examiner in clinical and preventive medicine was particularly interested in tropical diseases and gave me a thorough going-over on rinderpest or cattle plague. This suited me well because our Professor of Pathology, William Kearney, a flamboyant Corkman of outstanding charisma, had spent many years in Africa working on this disease. His lectures were riveting; he spoke from first hand experience of rinderpest and many other fascinating tropical diseases. To add to his dramatic presentation he seemed to have cultivated a tinge of Winston Churchill's tone and style. For a year I had sat captivated at his feet; he was my hero and my inspiration.

Therefore, amongst other things I managed to tell the examiner that rinderpest or cattle plague is a highly fatal disease that ravished the cattle populations of Europe, Asia and the Indian subcontinent during the greater part of the last two millennia; that it was eliminated from western Europe towards the end of the last century but still persisted in Asia and the Indian subcontinent; that at the turn of the century it made its way into East Africa for the first time ever and swept down like wildfire to South Africa where, there alone, it killed more than two million head of cattle during the course of a few years; and that it was eventually pushed back to East Africa. By 1943, unknown to me and while I was struggling to satisfy my examiner, rinderpest was being held with great difficulty only a few miles north of the Central Railway line that runs from Dar es Salaam, on the coast of the Indian Ocean, to Lake Tanganyika 700 miles to the west.

After further questioning about less exotic diseases his final question brought great comfort; he actually asked what I was going to do after the exams and strongly recommended the Colonial Veterinary Service. Little did I know that within eighteen months, at the age of twenty-three, I would be in charge of Tanganyika's Veterinary Laboratory at Mpwapwa, twelve miles north of the Central Railway line while the Acting Chief Veterinary Research Officer was on much needed leave in England. Such was the shortage of veterinary staff during the war years.

I was then ushered in to the examiner in surgery, a dapper Major in the Royal Army Veterinary Corps, poorly disguised in civilian clothes, the prescribed dress for visitors to neutral Ireland. The interview centred largely on the horse and ended on a relaxed note with some comments on the virtues of the mule in mountain warfare. Then, 'Well done young man, ever thought of joining the Corps?' The suggestion had come too late; the influence and advice of Professor Kearney had prompted me a few weeks earlier to submit a provisional application to the British Colonial Veterinary Services.

At the end of July I was called at very short notice for interview at the Colonial Office in London. Travel to Great Britain during the war was subject to the issuing of an Entry Permit by the United Kingdom Representative in Dublin and to securing a place on the London, Midland and Scottish Railway's Mail Boat to Holyhead. The formalities were cleared just in time to allow me and another would-be recruit, Desmond Hodgins (affectionately known as Hodge), one of my closest college friends, to arrive in London on the morning of the interview. It was just as hot as it can be in a London mid-summer heatwave. As we strolled up Park Street to identify the offices of the Director of Recruitment in preparation for our afternoon interviews, the heat in the confined street was almost intolerable, dressed as we were in our best Sunday suits and stiff white collars. We retreated to the shelter of a tree in Hyde Park to wait for the appointed time.

Hodge was a colourful, horsey character from the depths of County Clare who had travelled in his best tweed suit, complete with a single vent at the back, more suitable for a point to point race meeting in the winter than a London heatwave. He was famous for his colourful phrases and anecdotes about life in Clare. With perspiration trickling down his neck, even in the shade of our tree, he pulled his hand down over his luxuriant, jet-black moustache - a characteristic gesture that preceded many of his more dramatic pronouncements - and exclaimed, ' Jaze, I can't stand this heat; Lee, you are a cursed bloody man; you should never have dragged me over here to join the Colonial Service'. He was going to do his utmost to fail the interview just in case his resolve had weakened by the time he received an offer of appointment.

Travel-worn and perspiring, we were in no state to present ourselves for interview, so I persuaded Hodge to join me in gatecrashing the prestigious Dorchester Hotel, under the suspicious eye of an intimidating commissionaire. In the cool toilet we dried off and I removed my sodden detachable shirt collar and replaced it with a clean crisp one, which was sold with the shirt in those days before the advent of the washing machine. Meanwhile, Hodge had his tweed jacket off and, stripped to the waist, was having a refreshing sponge down in his characteristically vigorous way.

The tension and oppressive heat in the airless waiting room at 2 Park Street began to affect each of us in different ways. On my part, self-confidence was slipping away and passages from the recruitment manual flooded back. The Colonial Service required 'University men of character, ability and physical fitness'; spectacles were just acceptable but colour-blindness was out. Those suffering from an impediment of speech were tactfully, yet firmly, advised not to apply, 'because a disability of this kind is sometimes liable to become worse in the tropics and in any case must seriously hinder an officer in the performance of his duties, which may involve learning a native language'. One stumble from me, especially with an Irish accent, and I would be out!

In Hodge's case the trickling perspiration had irreversibly copper-fastened his resolve to screw-up the interview. The door suddenly opened and a member of the panel asked in a breezy voice, "Now, where's that man who hunts with the Scarteens?" and Hodge was shown in. Half an hour later a dejected candidate emerged. It subsequently transpired that his replies to the early questions, such as why he had applied for the Colonial Service, given in such a casual, jocular manner, and laced with amusing anecdotes had turned the interview into a refreshingly light-hearted affair for the panel. In due course, one of its more enthusiastic members began to describe some of the fascinating work waiting to be done in Africa. Hodge was enthralled but was so agitated at having blown the interview that he failed to realise that they were now selling the job to him! It seems the panel concluded that here was a self-confident, comical Irishman so full of the blarney that he could charm the hind legs off a donkey - just what was needed to keep everyone happy in a remote African outpost. The following year he was happily established in Northern Rhodesia in the process of acquiring his own string of race horses, far removed from the heat and humidity of the coast and, indeed, from the London heatwave.

All I can remember about my own interview was facing a panel of five which included a very elderly, tweedy gentleman immediately to the right of the chairman, an elbow on the table and an old-fashioned ear-trumpet grasped firmly in his hand. With the aperture pointing directly at my face, he asked why I had opted to apply for an appointment in the Colonial Service. As soon as I began to explain, concentrating on the importance of avoiding a stutter rather than on the amplitude of my reply, he cut me short, 'Can't hear a word you're saying, speak up there, speak up like a good fellow'. The chairman took it upon himself, probably out of kindness, to repeat the question and with a slight upward movement of one hand reminded me of the need for more volume. At that point, my immediate reaction was to say, 'Goodness only knows!' Needless to say, I did my best to give the right answers but, to me at least, they seemed utterly stupid as I heard them reverberating around the room.

In due course we were accepted, but the tropics were still a long way off for both of us. Despite the fact that the war was now at its height and there was a critical shortage of veterinary officers, particularly in Africa, the Colonial Office still persisted with a scheme initiated in 1929 which required veterinary recruits to take a course of instruction designed to develop further the scientific side of their education. Accordingly, we were notified that a postgraduate course was being arranged for us at Cambridge University. It was to be of three term's duration though we were warned that it might be curtailed if our services were urgently required 'in an emergency'. This was my first experience of the Colonial Office's administrators' stoical adherence to long-established procedures even while the bombs, flying bombs and eventually rockets were raining down on their very doorsteps. Admittedly, communications with the fifty or so separate governments distributed over the far flung two million square miles of the Colonial Empire were difficult and, at times impossible. On the other hand, the bureaucrats in London deserve credit for their unflinching conviction that no matter how long the war might last victory was inevitable and that standards had to be maintained come what may. Their lives in wartime London had been such a succession of emergencies for so long that they probably expected the governments they served overseas to cope equally well with their own particular emergencies.

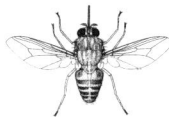

CHAPTER THREE

Cambridge Interlude

Fun, friendships and frustrations of College life in wartime Cambridge during studies prescribed by the Colonial Office. During sojourns in London the author experiences the stoicism of its inhabitants in the face of air raids by night and eventually flying bombs by day. The excitement of purchasing tropical outfit, following posting to Tanganyika.

B y the beginning of October Hodge and I had taken up residence at Emmanuel College, Cambridge. Although many of the undergraduates were obliged to stay in approved lodgings because a substantial area of the College had been handed over to the RAF, the Senior Tutor, Mr E. Welbourne, had kindly given us a fine suite of rooms in Front Square. The College had also conferred on us the privilege of M.A. status.

We were delighted to find that another pair of recruits to the Colonial Veterinary Service were also sharing similar rooms on our stair. Both of them, Dennis Walker and Ian Macadam, had just graduated from the Royal Veterinary College, London. As far as I am aware, the four of us as well as another more senior person who was posted overseas immediately, were the sum total of veterinary surgeons recruited during that year from Great Britain and Ireland to the entire Colonial Veterinary Service deployed throughout the two million square miles of the British Colonial Empire!

We were to each other as different as chalk is to cheese, yet our common identity within Emmanuel, as well as the fun and tribulations we shared together during the following nine months, established a warm bond of affection that continued throughout our lives. Dennis was a tall, good-looking young man who had spent his early years in Kenya where his father had been an administrative officer in the Veterinary

Department. He had a keen sense of humour and was fascinated by Hodge's and my Irishness. He enjoyed trying to mimic our accents to such an extent that I eventually taught him some greetings and phrases in Irish. One particularly meaningless phrase stuck and was always delivered with a laugh as his opening greeting on the many occasions when we met during the rest of his life. He also became a devotee of Myles na Gopaleen and was always hungry for fresh copy. But there was much more to Dennis than his sense of humour and I well remember some of the more serious philosophical and contemplative conversations we had over a pint of bitter or during long walks at the end of the day through Cambridge.

Although Mac, as we usually called Ian, had been born and educated in London his parents had a few years previously retired to Scotland, their native land, and Mac had become more Scottish than the Scots themselves. He was outstandingly the most enthusiastic and energetic member of our group and within our first few weeks at Cambridge he had joined so many of the university societies, such as boxing, ju-jitsu, horse riding and Scottish dancing, that I saw less of him than I did of Dennis and Hodge. However, when we were both posted to Tanganyika at the end of the Cambridge interlude, our friendship developed to the extent that I was his best man in his beloved Argyllshire in 1951.

We were delighted with the hospitality and friendliness of Emmanuel. The apartment that Hodge and I shared consisted of two bedrooms, a little kitchenette and a spacious sitting room. In the months ahead it was to be the scene of many parties including never-to-be-forgotten tea parties which were such a pleasant feature of college life, especially on wet, winter afternoons when the bitterly cold winds drove rain across the flat countryside between Cambridge and the North Sea beyond the Fens. More than fifty years later I can still hear Hodge entertaining our many English friends, as we sat around the open fire toasting muffins, with his stories about rural life in his beloved Clare: 'Did I ever tell you about the notorious widow woman of Cahermoore who took the ashplant to a randy insurance collector who tried to combine business with pleasure?'

At the beginning of term we were summoned by our tutor in the School of Agriculture to be informed about our course of study. We were to attend an extensive series of lectures on animal science including animal nutrition, animal production, genetics, breeding and artificial insemination. To expose us to more specific veterinary subjects we were to take lectures and practicals at the Molteno Laboratories of Parasitology and undertake a small research project under a supervisor at the Institute of Animal Pathology. It all looked very exciting. Most of our time was to be spent at the Downing Site within a stone's throw of Emma (Emmanuel). Sadly, disillusionment followed by depression crept in and deepened as the term progressed. The animal science lectures were for undergraduates and merely repeated those we had taken during our five years of veterinary training. The veterinary institute was rather rundown due to the exigencies of the war; consequently, each of our research projects was slow to start, half-hearted, rather pointless and largely unsupervised due to the shortage of scientific staff.

However, our weekly sessions at the Molteno were fun and more satisfying, thanks to the selfless dedication of our teacher Dr Tate, a rather self-conscious, gentle man of small stature, originally from Dublin. Everything about the Molteno was small and neat: the building itself; its labs; to a noticeable extent, its staff; and sadly, even the experimental animals with which we were obliged to work. Our teacher designed a course in experimental parasitology exclusively for us. He was a world authority on malaria of the canary which, presumably, was being used as a model for the study of the disease in humans. The disease was becoming immensely important as the war moved deeper and deeper into the tropics. He was always visibly embarrassed when he announced, with a nervous clearing of the throat, that the afternoon's exercise would deal with a protozoan parasite of the kidney of the frog, or perhaps the intestine of the mouse. He would always apologise, again with a slight cough, that it would be only of indirect veterinary interest. The confinement of our studies to small laboratory animals was admittedly a bit uninspiring for young vets hardly dry behind the ears and rearing to go in their chosen profession.

But our interest in the course soared every time we turned, wide-eyed, and with almost audible intakes of breath, to stare at Doris, the stunning little laboratory attendant - tailor-made for the Molteno in terms of size - as she glided demurely into the lab, balancing four enamel trays, each containing the limp carcass of an unfortunate little frog or mouse.

During the early sessions I am sure we all fantasized secretly about Doris but this was brought to an abrupt end when we learnt that Mac, a man of action, had lost no time in inviting her around to his rooms for tea. Thereafter, the rest of us had to be content with the dubious satisfaction of extracting microscopic parasites from the corpses of innocent little creatures while Mac bore an air of smug contentment during the exercises and was invariably first out, presumably to put the kettle on for another cosy little tea party. Dennis, his room-mate and a gentleman to the core, did not intrude; instead he joined us in our rooms and remained patiently with us long after the last of our toasted muffins had been consumed, until we heard the light tread of departing feet on the landing below.

Life in Cambridge, even in wartime, was a fascinating experience socially and before long we were, individually or collectively, involved in an extraordinary variety of clubs - my own favourite athletic activity being boxing. But all around us were the ever-present reminders that we were in the middle of a terrible war: queues at the butcher's, baker's and fishmonger's; painstaking efforts to charm a few cigarettes or currant buns from under the counter; the hoarding of a tin of sardines, and a cake or two from home for the next party in the rooms; National Dried Egg for a leathery omelette when we missed a square meal in Hall. The College Buttery did yeoman service in providing breakfast and dinner in Hall. The system involved handing over one's precious ration book at the beginning of term. No doubt this effected an economy in scale with the result that the meals were both adequate and satisfying. Nevertheless, it was always a pleasure to be asked, due to the shortage of labour, to take a turn at washing up the mountains of dirty dishes after dinner for a reward of a second helping behind the scenes! The minute butter ration and a small proportion of the sugar allowance was handed over by the Buttery every week to each individual for safe keeping and I can still see students and staff scurrying across Front Square for breakfast in Hall, clutching their little jars of these priceless commodities.

As the cold winds so characteristic of a Cambridge winter took hold, the minor deprivations associated with the food shortages reminded us of how trivial they were compared with their root cause, the Battle of the Atlantic, in which the Allies were only then beginning to get the upper hand. Even so, during 1943 the Germans built 283 new submarines of which an average of 212 were at sea, and by the end of that year 20 to 25 new subs were leaving German shipyards every month. Efforts to starve Britain out were still very much in progress. Equally provoking to one's conscience was the periodic droning overhead of huge formations of Flying Fortresses on their dangerous journeys to the carpet bombing of German cities from their bases on the flat land of the Eastern Counties, as were the truckloads of GIs that swept into Cambridge every weekend.

Our only contribution to all of this was manning the College Fire Brigade, an extension of the Auxiliary Fire Service. As the end of term approached our daily round of undergraduate lectures and irrelevant research exercises seemed embarrassingly out of place. At Christmas, in frustration, I wrote to the Colonial Office explaining that there was really no course for us at Cambridge and asked to be posted overseas straight away or, failing that, be allowed to join the Royal Army Veterinary Corps. In due course I received a courteous letter from London that urged me to devote myself to the subjects laid down in 'the course' but also informed me that I was free to study any other subject in which I was particularly interested during hours left vacant in the curriculum. I was assured that, with the wisdom of hindsight, I would eventually realise how valuable 'the course' had been. Subsequently I had to agree that the three terms at Cambridge, if not 'the course', had been well worthwhile!

With an easier conscience I drifted away from the more irrelevant undergraduate lectures and, for starters, sat at the feet of an excellent, elderly teacher in the Department of Anthropology. The class attending his fascinating course in primitive religions almost doubled in membership when the four of us were admitted! His accounts of some extraordinary customs and cures based on sympathetic magic persisting in remote parts of the Fens were almost as entertaining and not unlike some of Hodge's anecdotes about County Clare. As there was little, if any, opportunity to specialise in a veterinary discipline at Cambridge it seemed reprehensible not to take the opportunity to broaden our education when there was such quality available; before long I was attending lectures in psychology, sociology, and economics given by scholars of international repute. I also spent many happy hours in the University Library retracing the steps of Livingstone, Stanley, Burton and Speke, and other early explorers of Africa. What a joy it was a year later, following my posting to Mpwapwa, to know that this was one of the villages through which Stanley had passed seventy-three years earlier in his search for Livingstone, and to see the very tree under which he had camped, precisely as I had seen it in Stanley's *Through the Dark Continent* all the way back at Cambridge. In those times Africa and, in particular, remote villages like Mpwapwa were light years away in another world compared with the Africa of today's beach holidays and conducted tours of the Serengeti. The hackneyed phrase 'it's a small world' meant much more then than it does now!

Towards the end of term, as one approached the 'Backs' from the University Library, one began to see Cambridge coming into its best. How beautiful it was during a calm, sunny, spring day: the gently flowing river, fringed with weeping willows pushing out their delicate green leaves, reflecting the graceful arches of the bridges; isolated trees on the lawn sloping up to the colleges rising out of yellow carpets of daffodils. Removed as it was from the bustle of the town beyond the colleges, the peace and tranquillity made one feel that one was seeing the scene as it had been seen by many generations long gone. On one occasion, when I was lost in one of my reveries, a canoe lazily paddled by a pair of students glided into view with scarcely a ripple on the dead calm surface of the river. The canoe drew my eye across the river to a naval officer reclining on a bench, contentedly puffing his pipe as he too watched its slow passage. I was abruptly brought back to earth - it was 1944 and there was a war on.

It was tempting to stay on at Cambridge over the vacation to enjoy the quietness that descended on Emma after the noisy undergraduates had left. We were virtually on half-pay, however, and sheer necessity drove the four of us to seek locums wherever the fancy took us. For some long-forgotten reason I chose the East End of London where I found myself in charge of a branch practice for dogs and cats. I have two outstanding memories which reflect the circumstances of the time as well as the warmth and friendliness of London's East Enders. It was a live-in job and the ménage consisted of a youngish secretary cum cook/housekeeper/ general factotum who ran the show, a teenage girl who looked after the animals, and some veterinary locums who came and went. It was long before the days of mixed-sex living but we were all happily accommodated in the little terraced house. London had been relatively quiet for some time but almost immediately after my arrival there was a series of night raids. At the time the Germans were dropping whistling bombs to terrify the civilian population and I have to admit that they succeeded wonderfully well with me initially. Nevertheless, a few sessions in the flimsy shelter under the stairs in pleasantly close proximity to my cheerfully pragmatic, well-seasoned East End girlfriends soon enabled me to join in their detached speculation as to precisely where the last bomb had fallen.

One night there was an horrendous explosion disagreeably close by. The following evening as I walked along a nearby road towards the Underground there was a new rubble-strewn gap, like a missing tooth, in a terrace of houses. An elderly couple had been killed outright. Details were available from the corner shop but there was little talk about it; just another incident past which people had hurried on their way to work that morning. How difficult it is for the present generation of young people, as they watch soap operas of today's Londoners, to comprehend just what the Londoners of those times sustained with such valour during five years of bombs, doodle-bugs and eventually rockets.

A somewhat less threatening incident was the saga of the lost cat. Within the first few days of my arrival an elderly widow brought in her treasured companion: a rather unpleasant tabby cat with a nasty abscess above the eye. The owner reluctantly allowed us to keep it in for a few days. Two or three days later we found, to our horror, the cat had escaped; it was gone despite having been securely caged within our 'escape-proof' cattery! When the lady called for her next progress report I came clean and explained 'Well actually . . . I do not quite know how but - it has escaped'. Her reaction was dreadful! I eventually got a word in and introduced a glimmer of hope by assuring her that we were searching all the nooks and crannies on the premises. Next morning my colleagues joined me to explain that cats were rather like pigeons, they have a strong homing instinct, and in the unlikely event that her pet was not still on our premises she should let us know as soon as it made its way back to her. Thereafter, every morning my heart sank as I opened the waiting room door to see her sitting there, *sans* cat, poised for yet another difficult conversation. In due course, our conversations became less focused, cups of tea crept in and more general topics were introduced. Eventually, we learnt quite a lot about each other's families and talked of my plans for the future. On the final day of my locum she brought in a photo of her late husband and a recent one of her son who had just been posted to Italy. She wished us all well as she left and presumed, almost as an after-thought, that there was no news of the cat. There she went, her original resentment forgotten, just a kind, lonely old lady who had just lost her last remaining companion. Nowadays the benefits a household pet brings to the well-being and health of the frail elderly are better understood.

Back at Cambridge there were signs that the war was building up to something very, very big, yet security was so effective that the civilian population had no idea whatsoever that the invasion of Europe would begin only a hundred miles to the south less than two months later. For some time huge dumps of artillery shells, boxes of ammunition and other armaments, quite unattended, had been accumulating on grass verges of minor country roads not being used by the County Agricultural Committees for growing wheat and barley.

During this build-up the long-established traditions of Cambridge, such as May Week with its May Ball, all night parties, and the May Bumps on the river were faithfully adhered to though they reflected only a little of their former glory. Then on 6 June the momentous announce-ment on the radio told us that D-Day had arrived and the Allied Forces were already landing on the Normandy beaches. A letter I wrote to my family in Dublin illustrated the strict security that existed between the United Kingdom and Ireland throughout the war. All letters going and coming across the Irish Sea carried a seal stating that they had been 'Opened by the Examiner'. In my letter of 6 June I merely stated that the first thing we knew about the 'European business' was what they had, no doubt, heard simultaneously on the BBC. So conditioned were we by the ubiquitous propaganda notices, such as 'Idle Talk Costs Lives', that one gave no details.

Trinity Term at Cambridge ended a few days later after many touching farewell parties followed by the sad noise of students trundelling trolley-loads of suitcases and boxes out of Emma, in many cases for the last time. The four of us were kindly allowed to remain on to use the College as our base until we received our overseas postings from the Colonial Office. The intervening time was pleasantly spent on a locum in farm animal practice with Ron Webber and his wife Beryl who were new found friends at nearby Royston. Early in July I was informed that I was being posted to Tanganyika, as was Mac. Hodge was destined for Northern Rhodesia, while Dennis, who had spent most of his childhood in Kenya and spoke Kiswahili, strangely was posted to Nigeria in West Africa. Perhaps it was because of rinderpest that as many as three of us were allocated to the East Coast, but why not poor Dennis with his Kiswahili? We suspected that the future course of our lives had been decided either in alphabetical order or by the prick of a pin! It surprised me to learn that I was unlikely to sail before mid-October - a foretaste of the difficulties of overseas travel during wartime.

With my posting settled there was business to attend to in London with Griffiths McAlister, the famous 'Purveyor of Complete Outfits, General Agents and Taxidermists' of 10 Warwick Street W.1. Even at the height of the war, Griffiths McAlister could still supply: 'small egg cups for tropical eggs'; mosquito boots; field service uniforms and safari jackets complete with red felt spine-pads 'to protect one from the deleterious effects of the tropical sun'; ugly Wallesey sun helmets curving down over the back of the neck for further protection; elegant portable safari baths sufficiently light for head porterage; hurricane lamps and much more. 'How exciting! This is for real!' Number ten Warwick Street was the gateway to Africa.

There was now other excitement in the streets of London. A week after D-Day Hitler launched his first secret weapon, the V1 Flying Bombs or 'Doodle Bugs', specifically targeted on London to terrorise the population. They came in at an altitude of about 3,000 feet, carrying a ton of explosives at 375 mph. During the following three months 7,500 were launched but they were easy prey for fighter aircraft and AA guns; many exploded in mid-air with the result that only half of this number fell on London. Nevertheless, in London 25,000 houses were destroyed and 6,000 people were killed. Despite that, they were not too frightening as one walked about London during daylight. On the contrary, they were somewhat entertaining because, coming in at such a low altitude, one could see them clearly and hear the drone of their jet engines. Provided the sound continued one could relax and, with luck, watch them pass overhead. On the other hand if the engine cut out there was a mad rush for cover. In general, Londoners continued to go about their life as calmly as ever. Air raid alerts for the Doodle Bugs were of such long duration that one forgot whether the previous siren had been an 'alert' or an 'all clear'. For clarification one could check the notice displayed outside entrances to the Underground as the crowds flowed in and out about their business, largely unconcerned as to whether it was 'all clear' or 'alert'. After three months the situation became much more sinister when V2 rockets began to arrive. Their speed was such that the explosion was heard first, followed by the deafening roar of their arrival.

Restrictions on travel to Ireland necessitated Hodge and me making advanced arrangements for obtaining permits to cross the Irish Sea. In Hodge's case difficulties arose which necessitated delicate negotiaton on the part of my intrepid friend to prevent inflicting a nervous breakdown on his bride-to-be, Hazel. The previous January he had found a job in Cambridge for his fiancée which was of sufficient importance to justify the authorities issuing a travel permit, whereupon he had induced her to leave the peace and plenty of County Clare to join him. Preliminary phone calls to London failed to yield a permit for her return to Ireland. So after several highly-charged emotional scenes with Hazel, involving much downward stroking of the moustache by a contemplative Hodge, he set off early one morning in a grim, purposeful manner for a face-to-face encounter with the authorities in London. Very late that night he burst into our rooms greatly elated and explained (probably with a reference to those 'cursed bloody' people) that Hazel could under no circumstances travel to Ireland other than as his wife. Practical and resourceful as ever, and after much effort and expense, he had obtained a special marriage licence. Thereupon, he hurried off to tell Hazel that they were getting married the following morning if he could get an appointment for the purpose at the Registry Office.

Having been summarily appointed best man, I managed to secure the necessary appointment for two mornings hence. At the appointed time the wedding party, including Dennis and Mac, literally got on its bikes and cycled to the Registrar's Office. After quite a touching little ceremony and as the formal kiss was being exchanged, the fatherly Registrar turned discreetly to me and murmured that he needed seven shillings and six pence. To my dismay I discovered that I was short of a few bob, so the Registrar and I clustered around an obliging Dennis while we picked through the small change in his supplicating hands!

The wedding reception was unpretentious. We simply propped our bikes against the first pub, had a sandwich and toasted the happy couple with mild and bitter. A honeymoon was out of the question because Hazel, born of the Rectory, refused to regard the day's proceedings as a real marriage so the reasonably happy couple returned at nightfall to their respective lonely beds. Furthermore, we were all sworn to secrecy because, now that a travel permit was assured, Daddy was to do the proper job himself in complete ignorance of the couple's new marital status.

Back in Clare the wedding, attended by two bishops, other clergy and many relatives and friends, was a very formal, morning dress affair. The tight-lipped bride unashamedly used the present tense, instead of the past, when she assured her father in response to his solemn enquiry that she did, indeed, take this man to be her lawful wedded husband. Nevertheless, there was a tense moment for the otherwise happy couple when the congregation was asked '. . . if any man can show any just cause why they may not lawfully be joined together, let him now speak, or else hereafter forever hold his peace'. However, while the previous best man and another guest from Cambridge had not shown their hand before the ceremony, they were both quite satisfied in the circumstances that there was no 'just cause' to screw the whole thing up at that stage!

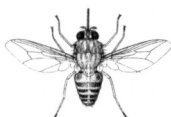

CHAPTER FOUR

Waiting for a Ship

Pleasant time, mainly on locums, first in Ireland then in England. Suddenly summoned to a bizarre interview in London with the Duke of Devonshire, Parliamentary Undersecretary of State for the Colonies. An aborted departure from Glasgow emphasised the importance of security (Careless Talk Costs Lives).

My marching orders had been accompanied by an official booklet describing 'Living Conditions in Tanganyika Territory'. Back in Ireland I had ample time to study its contents and I am afraid the health risks it outlined were accepted as gospel truth by my sister Anna with whom I shared most things. It was she who faithfully filed all my subsequent letters in anticipation, I suspect, that each one as it arrived was likely to be the last!

The booklet demonstrated how remote and misunderstood East Africa was in those days. The perceived effects of tropical climates were highly subjective and at points bordered on fantasy. The climate of the coastal region of Tanganyika was believed to bring about 'a gradual lack of tone' which was cumulative, with the result that prolonged residence 'tends to result in a gradual deterioration in mental and physical energy'. The effects were supposed to be decidedly more obvious in women, the unmarried and sedentary workers than outdoor types. Even if one had the good fortune to be stationed at bracing, high altitudes there was a catch; 'lengthy residence at these altitudes was apt to produce nervous manifestations'!

In general, personality seemed to be the answer. 'The best type of individual is one possessed of an even temper, who takes a cheerful outlook on life, and is not easily disturbed by reverses. Those subject to fits of depression, violent temper, nervous and unbalanced types are unsuitable for the tropics'. Surely, such 'types' should have been told so the previous year prior to interview, when the unfortunate colour-blind, stuttering candidates were being warned off!

Tanganyika did not seem to be a great place either for the family man; even the most even-tempered, cheery couples, undisturbed by 'reverses' might well have decided to remain childless after reading this literature. Those of their children who managed to survive various forms of enteritis and the effects of improper feeding would have very little to look forward to, oddly enough, after their fourth birthday! According to the booklet, 'After the fourth year climatic influences become more distinctly operative . . . It may be taken that the higher the temperature the more susceptible is the nervous system to external stimuli, which may result in premature overgrowth of strength, an unbalanced metabolism, nerve exhaustion, anaemia, malnutrition of the organs and muscular structure, and contact with native servants may promote the establishment of a mental attitude, processes of ideation and thought foreign to children born, bred and educated in England.'

Incidentally, in this official document 'England' was used exclusively for Great Britain. One came from and went to England; never to the United Kingdom, or to Scotland, Wales or Northern Ireland. One should bring some of the clothes one wore in England; tobacco was cheaper than in England; hospitals for Europeans in the larger centres were OK, they had English nursing staff. Coming from the Irish Free State this passed over me until I eventually learnt that some two-thirds of the members of the Colonial Service, particularly in the professional departments who actually ran the Colonial Empire, were Scottish, Welsh and Irish. The political officers, such as Provincial and District Commissioners and District Officers, generally referred to as the Administration, were in the main arts graduates of Cambridge, Oxford and oddly, Trinity College Dublin.

On a more serious note, the booklet's references to the precautions that had to be taken against tropical diseases such as malaria, typhoid, cholera, bilharzia, tick fever and sleeping sickness were telling and helpful especially at that time when therapeutic treatments, if any, for these and many other tropical diseases, left much to be desired. In those days quinine was the only treatment for malaria. It was a very unpleasant drug and towards the end of a course one became deaf and remained so for several days. Furthermore, it was not suitable as a prophylactic other than in exceptional circumstances. Consequently, prevention consisted of protecting oneself against mosquito bites. Therefore, in malarious areas it was almost obligatory after sundown to wear mosquito boots, which were rather like elegant wellies reaching to the knee. Ladies put on long dresses to the ankle and men changed into long-sleeved shirts and full-length trousers. These precautions against mosquitoes were taken seriously because in the absence of today's synthetic anti-malarials, the disease was prevalent and its dreadful complication, blackwater fever, was not uncommon.

Old colonials who lived through that strict regimen of post-sundown attire tend to be dismayed (probably some of them are just titillated!) by the exposed limbs and bare backs of the present generation of whites as they gather to sip their pre-prandial sundowners. Perhaps the current, rapidly-spreading distribution of drug-resistant malaria parasites which have evolved as a result of the misuse of these excellent drugs will resurrect the old reliable mosquito boots if new drugs or adequately effective insect-repellents are not forthcoming.

At the beginning of October (just as I was completing a locum for Trevor Scott in Bray, Co.Wicklow) I received a most courteous letter from the Private Secretary to His Grace the Duke of Devonshire, Parliamentary Undersecretary of State for the Colonies. It stated that His Grace 'would much like to see you before you sail to take your new appointment in Tanganyika'. I was greatly surprised, perhaps a little apprehensive, as to why he should wish to see an inconspicuous youngster like me. In any event, it was high time to go to London to complete my business with Messrs Griffiths McAlister.

On arrival at the Colonial Office in Downing Street, His Grace's Private Secretary graciously ushered me into the ante-room adjacent to the Duke's apartment but, before withdrawing to announce my arrival, she gave me no inkling of the nature of the business at hand. On her return she told me that His Grace would see me now, whereupon she swung the door open and to my astonishment revealed the longest study I had ever seen. There, in the distance, sat His Grace behind a massive desk. I can still remember my concern that I must not trip as I strode over the thick carpet on my way to meet the second-in-command of the huge colonial empire. This was big stuff!

I was received like an equal, 'How good of you to come, Lee', or words to that effect, as I was offered a chair at my side of the desk. A relaxed conversation, over a cigarette proffered from the then conventional heavy silver cigarette box, ensued. All I can recall is that at one stage he mentioned that every effort was made to deal justly with the citizens of the colonies and that everyone, from the highest to the lowest, had the right to appeal in serious cases through him to the Privy Council. He picked up a document with which he was dealing and pointed to a particular passage without, of course, mentioning the appellant's name. As I craned over the wide desk he invited me around to his side. By then I had been made to feel so much at ease with this gracious gentleman that I had to check a spontaneous reaction to put an arm around his shoulder as we studied the document together. Shortly thereafter, he thanked me again for calling and wished me well.

I never learnt why I was singled out to be privileged in this way. Maybe it was considered of some importance to show the kinder face of the colonial empire's establishment to a sample of Irish recruits. If so, a more genuine gentleman than His Grace could not have been chosen to fill that role.

There was no question of returning to Dublin at this stage. I had already said my sad farewells to my family, and the memory of my two sisters, Molly and Anna, waving from the end of Kingstown (now Dun Laoghaire) Pier until they were just visible, slender as matchsticks, on the distant horizon was still uppermost in my mind. It was a particularly sad parting because over the years they had slipped their young brother most of the cash for such luxuries as the hiring of tails and white ties for the annual dress dances of the Veterinary College and sister institutions and for courting girlfriends in general. One could not in all conscience extract funding for such extra-curricular activities from my generous parents whose business was hard-pressed by the exigencies of the war. Furthermore, none of us had any idea how many years would pass before our next meeting. In any event, I had to hold myself in readiness to report to my ship at short notice and that meant waiting in England because of the difficulties of travel to and from Ireland.

My good friends near Cambridge, the Webbers, with whom I had done weekend locums while at Emmanuel, had by then accepted me as a member of the family and invited me to make their house a home from home. It was a happy arrangement. Locums and assistants were in very short supply and Ron was run off his feet, so he was delighted to have me to help out with calls. Poor Beryl, who was expecting her first baby, was also hard-pressed because, apart from being unable to get domestic help, she was also tied to the telephone and consequently to the house. We even tried to get my mother to recruit a maid for her in Ireland! Despite that it was a house full of laughter with many hilarious moments. The excitement they shared with me in waiting each day for the arrival of sailing instructions was also touching. It proved to be the start of a life-long friendship.

After just over a week, a large envelope arrived containing labels marked DESTINATION 5. My destination was Durban and I was to proceed by train to a shipping agent in Glasgow to join a ship that was to sail five days later. I was instructed not to disclose the sailing date of the ship or its destination to anybody. Meanwhile, I had to shoot down post-haste to Griffiths McAlister in London with the labels for my heavy boxes which had to be despatched to Glasgow immediately. Security was tight and the documentary information informed passengers that 'Careless Talk Costs Lives'. They were warned against mentioning before, during or after their voyage any information regarding ports of call, destinations, routes, escorts, convoys, defensive armaments or casualties. Diaries were not to be kept and cameras were to be handed over to the Commander of the vessel on boarding. Officialdom's organisation was superb and these instructions were taken seriously by all concerned rather than being treated dismissively as red tape; such was society's spirit of cooperative obedience during the war.

Passengers were also instructed to take with them their national registration identity cards, clothing coupons, ration books and gas masks either for inspection or surrender at the port of embarkation. The thought of surrendering those precious possessions, combined with the above-mentioned warnings, brought home the reality that one was about to cast off the warm, comfortable network of friendships in England and enter a hostile, unknown world of convoys out there in the cold darkness of the advancing winter.

After another sad farewell, this time at Royston Station at the crack of dawn, it was a dreary twelve-hour journey in grossly overcrowded trains to Glasgow via London and Edinburgh. Early next morning a large number of sodden passengers accumulated in pouring rain with their piles of heavy baggage labelled with various destination numbers in a decrepit, long-forgotten warehouse somewhere down the Clyde. When all were gathered we were informed that our vessel, a brand new Liberty Ship, of the type being mass-produced in the United States by a process involving welding instead of riveting, had just failed its trials. We were told to go home pending further instructions.

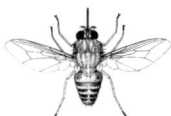

CHAPTER FIVE

Liverpool to Tanganyika:
Three Months in Wartime

A fascinating journey for six weeks on an old ship leaving Liverpool in a huge convoy, then steaming slowly across the cold Atlantic before heading south alone on the vast ocean visiting Ascension Island, Saint Helena, Cape Town, Port Elizabeth, East London and Durban. From there on to Beira, Zanzibar and, at last, Dar es Salaam.

A week later I was instructed to make my way to the Victoria Docks at Liverpool to board the *T 75* which was due to sail on 2 November. It was a happier experience than the previous one in Glasgow. We were taken by lighter to the *T 75* which was lying well out in the Mersey, barely visible in the fading light of a cold, winter afternoon. Not a light was showing in the blackout either on the ship or elsewhere. We subsequently learnt that it was an old ship with a speed of only 12 knots. It had been through the First World War and after a long career with the Shaw Saville Line plying mainly between the United Kingdom and Australia it was retrieved from a breaker's yard at Rosyth at the outbreak of the Second World War. It was then fitted with what looked like serviceable naval guns fore and aft and a battery of heavy rapid-fire anti-aircraft machine guns, known as Chicago Pianos, amidships. There were various rafts along the side of the promenade deck reminding us of the need for these armaments.

I was fortunate to be allocated a four-bunk cabin with three other passengers all bound for Tanganyika. Two were new recruits of about my own age. Jack was a boiler inspector from the midlands of England who was to report in the first instance to the Railway Workshops at Dar es

Salaam. Beyond that he had little notion as to what life held for him there. The other recruit, Owen, was an accountant from Belfast who was fortunate in knowing that he was to be stationed in the delightfully cool Usambara Highlands in Northern Tanganyika near Tanga. Our other travelling companion, Charles, was a District Officer returning from his first home leave having already completed a long tour of service. We were fortunate to have his company because he readily became a fascinating source of information about the country and its language (Kiswahili). Little did we know that we were to be thrown together for the next six weeks in this cramped cabin all the way to Durban, from where we would continue our journey to arrive in Tanganyika after yet another six weeks, and still the best of friends. We were allowed access to the baggage room and a hold to check that our loads had arrived. Having last seen them in the decrepit warehouse in Glasgow I marvelled at the efficiency of the Crown agents when I saw them neatly stacked away, once again on their long journey to DESTINATION 5. Other passengers were checking baggage marked DESTINATION 1, 2, 3, 4 or 5. Over the next few days as folk got to know each other the numbers were deciphered as Ascension Island, Cape Town, Port Elizabeth, East London and Durban. At that point we were unaware that we would also have the fun of a day ashore at the island of Saint Helena. Quite a trip lay ahead for us!

Even though the docks were only two or three hundred yards away we were already in a different world; a world of plenty already far from wartime England. No more rubbery omelettes or scrambled egg made from National Dried Egg, no more thin scrapes of precious butter on the morning toast without long-forgotten marmalade. I can still remember the contrast of sitting down to the first dinner - roast duck served with real orange sauce, followed amongst other delicacies by a fruit salad containing oranges, bananas and melon, all unseen since 1939. I can still see the pineapple decorating the centre of the table. Presumably the fruit had been taken on board during the *T 75*'s homeward voyage.

After a day or two we moved purposefully out of the Mersey well into the open sea where we joined several other ships, corvettes and warships. Each day the number of vessels grew. As each merchantman arrived it was shepherded into its proper station and, in due course, a huge convoy was formed that stretched as far as the eye could see in the dull November light.

Eventually, the convoy appeared to be on its way. Each morning my cabin mates and I, who were by now close companions, joined a group of fellow travellers on deck to speculate as to our progress. Inevitably, there were wise guys that argued vociferously about our precise location. Three days into our journey one of the amateur navigators was convinced that we were now in the Atlantic far out from Donegal, having passed through the North Channel, but another argued that we had left the Irish Sea via Saint George's Channel and the Fastnet was far behind us. These heated discussions were rather pointless. After all, one seldom got a glimpse of blue skies, far less the sun by day or the stars by night as we ploughed through the cold, grey overcast sea. Happily, on this particular occasion the sun broke through. There, clearly visible on the distant horizon, was the unmistakable peak of the Sugar Loaf Mountain that lies just south of Dublin. What a joy it was to see it again so soon after my sad farewells! Our crestfallen navigators fell silent as it dawned on us that we had been going round and round in circles for days and were still less than a hundred miles from Liverpool. Remarkably one of them had the misfortune to be called Henry and, needless to say, 'the Navigator' was added and it stuck. Shortly thereafter, the convoy set forth purposefully at a quicker pace for the Atlantic, but not all that fast because its speed was limited by the maximum speed of the slowest ship, which may have been the *T 75*'s twelve knots.

Henry, being a good-natured individual, soon recovered his self-confidence and kept us informed as we steamed across the Atlantic keeping stations faithfully with each of the four nearest ships lying ahead, astern, to starboard and to port. When we went on deck each morning it was somehow comforting to see each of these reliable old companions in precisely the same position in which we had left them the previous evening before the fading light ushered in the blackout that eventually obscured them from view. The way in which the ships kept their stations in such difficult circumstances was a tribute to the skills of the Merchant Navy.

This was not the time of year to linger on deck. Below decks a pleasant routine evolved which revolved around hearty breakfasts, morning coffees, lunches and five-course dinners followed by a ritual cigar and South African brandy with my now almost inseparable cabin mates. The meals were separated by nothing more serious than housey-housey, betting on the distance we had travelled during the past twenty-four hours as determined by the log, which was trailed in the water from the ship's stern, and chatting with new-found friends. This was the life of Riley compared with the austerity of home, the memory of which was steadily receding far beyond the wake of the *T 75*.

One morning when we went on deck for the usual pre-breakfast breath of air we were shocked to find that the *T 75* was completely on its own. We were heading south across an empty sea. It transpired that we had been shepherded almost to the coast of North America as far as possible from the dangerous waters of West Africa where the German submarines were still particularly active. From then on we became more conscious of the risks at sea. We were now zigzagging and boat drills were more frequent. Not all of the drills were for practice and from time to time flotsam was sighted bobbing up and down on the distant waves reminding us that sinkings did occur and also that U-boats used the cover of wreckage to conceal their periscopes from approaching ships. On such occasions, when we reached our boat stations, we were entertained by the manning of the forward gun and the firing of a salvo of shells at the distant wreckage. Fortunately, all of these alarms proved to be false though they did bring us up sharply to our vulnerability and to the fact that we were entirely alone on our own isolated sweep of the vast ocean.

As each day passed the weather became warmer, the sky bluer and the sea smoother. Just as the coming of spring changes the whole environment our steady passage southwards had the same effect. The occasional flying fish was spotted surfacing from the bow wave; their numbers steadily increased as if the word had gone around that the *T 75* was back and more and more wanted to escort their old friend into warmer waters. Nets for deck tennis appeared, white lines were re-painted and quoits brought out. Tweed jackets and mufflers were left below and suddenly the ship's officers appeared in white tropical uniform, short-sleeved and bare-kneed, as if in holiday mood after the formal navy blue. This was accompanied by the rigging of a very functional canvas swimming pool over one of the holds. In due course Father Neptune, complete with long beard and trident, came aboard as we crossed the Equator and soaped, shaved and ducked anybody his assistants could grab who were crossing the line for the first time. From then on life on deck was idyllic: friendships became more relaxed; life stories were exchanged over Tom Collins and Pimms; love affairs, their numbers limited only by the availability of unattached females (of any age), flourished. Two engagements were celebrated and one marriage was performed by the Captain before we reached Cape Town.

A day or so after crossing the Equator we must have been near the coast of Brazil. We then headed east for some days to Ascension Island where we dropped anchor and took off two Cable and Wireless men who had been on that barren peak for two years. Its isolation was awe-inspiring and the only features to commend it were the colourful tip of the peak brushed green by passing clouds and the shoals of a wide variety of brilliantly coloured tropical fish that entertained us as we lined the decks of the *T 75*. We shouted our goodbyes to the two replacements who were lowered to the lighter with their baggage marked DESTINATION 1. They must have been hand-picked to tolerate each other's company in the loneliness of that peak separated, as they were, from their nearest neighbours more than 800 miles away to the south on the island of Saint Helena. Some days later we anchored off Saint Helena to take on fresh water and coal. That gave us time to go ashore and visit Napoleon's house on that fascinating island. What a joy it was to stretch our legs on dry land after precisely three weeks at sea and to see bananas growing at the roadside! On our sail down to Cape Town with Christmas only a few weeks away a number of us got into a routine of snuggling down for a singsong on the upper deck warming our backs in the cool night air against the hot funnel. Ever since then, coming up to Christmas when 'Silent Night' is sung, I am back with my friends on the deck, looking towards the Southern Cross in the cloudless, starry sky, conscious of the gentle rise and fall of the bows and the sound and smell of steam escaping from a nearby pipe.

Another week saw us sailing into Cape Town where our DESTINATION 2 friends bid us farewell as the rest of us set off to climb Table Mountain and to experience the never-to-be-forgotten smell of the pine resin in the sunshine as we ascended the mountain. One had to climb all the way up in those days, for it was long before the advent of the cable car. The other memorable smell was that of a bewildering variety of fruit permeating the ship following our return from compulsive shopping sprees at the fruit markets. Having parted with so many friends at Cape Town and a few more at Port Elizabeth and East London, the cramped conditions aboard the scruffy old *T 75* began to lose their appeal and my cabin mates and I were now itching to get to Durban and hopefully on to Tanganyika without further delay. We eventually disembarked at Durban almost six weeks after leaving London.

Durban was a wonderfully luxurious interlude between the confined life aboard the *T 75* and the simple, unsophisticated life waiting for me in Tanganyika where the acquisition of a short wave radio, working off a twelve-volt car battery, and a refrigerator powered by paraffin oil were to be major breakthroughs which had to wait for another fifteen months. Durban itself had its own contrasts: high-rise, luxury hotels, spacious tin-roofed bungalows and thatched mud huts; smart cocktail bars for the whites and dreadful 'beer gardens' for the blacks, more like cages for wild animals than bars; chauffeur-driven American cars parked on Marine Parade beside rickshaws pulled by handsome, immensely entertaining Zulus in full war dress; empty benches at railway stations reserved for whites while crowds of blacks had to stand. While most of my shipmates and I were disturbed and, at times, shocked by the colour bar, I am afraid these sentiments did not interfere with our enjoyment of the luxury hotels on Marine Parade in which we were billeted, or the pleasures of surfing in the Indian Ocean just a few steps beyond the other side of the road.

Immediately after Christmas, those of us bound for East Africa boarded the *Straat Soenda*, a small Dutch freighter that presumably was overseas or else had managed to escape, as did Queen Wilhelmina, her government and much of the merchant fleet, when the Netherlands was overrun by German tanks and paratroopers during the course of only five days in May 1940.

Our circle of friends was now reduced to a small group destined to disembark at Zanzibar and Dar es Salaam, some 2,000 miles to the north. Life settled down to a rather dull routine after the fleshpots of Durban. Being south of the Equator we were in the middle of the hot season and it was getting hotter every day. Two days later we arrived off the port of Beira, Portuguese East Africa (now Sofala, Mozambique) and to our dismay we dropped anchor and waited for another two days. All we could see across the deadly calm, lifeless sea was a long, flat palm-fringed coastline with a few tin-roofed buildings and some occasional cars looking like little Dinky toys, passing to and fro. The sky was overcast and the heat oppressive. After two long days a ship emerged from the estuary and as it passed we were all surprised to see that it was, of all things, Swiss registered. We moved in and tied-up to the vacant jetty on the river at the end of a railway that runs to Zimbabwe and there links up with South Africa and Zambia. Almost immediately, a gang of bare-footed Africans swarmed aboard and began to unload sugar from the forward hold. There was not a breath of air as we stood watching from the shelter of a canopy stretched over the deck and even in that shade our clammy shirts stuck to the chest. The temperature was an horrendous 120° F and humid as well. Needless to say, sweat poured down the backs of the stevedores as they struggled with the bags in the depth of the sweltering hold. Normally, a gang of Africans swing into their work with a rousing chorus led by a happily extroverted leader. There was no singing on this occasion, it was just too hot; the work was done in deadly silence. At the end of the day, after they had dried themselves down with shirts made from sugar bags, we learnt that they received the princely sum of sixpence a day for their efforts. This was exploitation at its worst. We were shocked.

The walk towards the outskirts of Beira, through dead flat, low-lying terrain was literally not worth the sweat. We were dubiously rewarded by finding only a few decrepit shops whose unwelcoming, listless Portuguese proprietors seemed to have accepted that there was nothing better to do than lounge in front of their half-empty shelves in a state of suspended animation. I could not help feeling that the author of the Colonial Office's official booklet on living conditions in Tanganyika had passed this way. He was indeed right; the climate in the coastal region was believed to bring about 'a general lack of tone' which was cumulative, with the result that prolonged residence 'tends to result in general deterioration in mental and physical energy'. He had put it mildly, but these poor chaps probably hadn't had leave for twenty years, if ever. They had probably been born here.

Back on board the depression deepened and reached its nadir on New Year's Eve. The Ship's Officers threw a party on deck and the few women on board were kept busy dancing to the strains of guitars. With a surplus of men the drinking was extra and before long some of the sailors became maudlin, others footless. Towards midnight, one of the sailors and a young woman who had left her elderly parents at home in England in order to join her husband in Tanganyika and I, being more sober than the rest, drifted off to the Upper Deck to bring in the New Year together. Up there all attempts at gaiety petered out as we sat staring out into the darkness. My thoughts were thousands of miles away in front of a roaring fire of turf, previously dried out for the occasion, where my father with a glass of the hard stuff was toasting 'absent friends'. For the first time on my travels, I was acutely homesick. At long last the *Straat Soenda*'s siren heralded in the New Year. Tongue in cheek, we wished each other a Happy New Year. The sailor, head in hands and weeping gently, muttered that his young family was in occupied Java and scurried away below decks. Thereupon, the young wife began whimpering, put her arms around my shoulders and then followed him down the companionway. I said to myself, 'Janey Mack!' feeling hard done by; dammit, I had been left with nobody's shoulder to cry on! There was no future to speak of; we were all going to be stationed in Tanganyika's coastal zone. After all, had I not been warned? Already I could feel 'the general lack of tone' as my mental and physical energy drained away! I drifted off to my sticky, airless cabin. Air conditioning was unheard of in those days. We had another four days of abject boredom before departure. Beira was a dead loss!

Our next port of call was at Zanzibar for a three day stop. It was fun. As we dropped anchor not far from the sparklingly white Sultan's Palace an exciting smell of spices reached us from the shore. The brisk passage to and fro of Arab dhows under full sail told us that this was a place full of life and industry, as did the figures of turbaned Arabs and Africans striding smartly along the sea front. Almost immediately, a flotilla of small boats and lighters assembled alongside and customs and other officials began to set up their desks in the ship's dining room. Our cabin mate Charles had given us lessons in Kiswahili every day at the breakfast table for five weeks. As a result we could now carry on simple conversations between ourselves, so when I spotted an imposing African policeman at the immigration desk I elbowed my way through the crowd and greeted him with a well enunciated, '*Jambo Askari, habari za Zanzibar.*' To my surprise, I had to repeat it. Imagine my mortification when he courteously replied, 'Sorry Bwana, I no speak English!'

When we got ashore a group of us made for the market where we were intrigued by the displays of strange fish, pawpaw, mangoes, bananas, green-skinned oranges, grapefruit, sweet potatoes and much more that was strange to us. As we wandered around I noticed that we were being scrutinised at some distance by a European lady. Eventually she approached and engaged us in conversation. She explained that very few ships called now so it was a great pleasure to have visitors from the outside world. She invited us all to her house to meet her husband who was due home for lunch from the courthouse where he was Resident Magistrate. An opportunity to be invited into our first East African house was one not to be missed. We gladly meandered slowly, as one did in the midday heat, through the narrow streets with their elaborately carved doors, so typical of Zanzibar, to her house. There we were served precious cold beers by dignified servants resplendent in long white robes, known as *kanzus*, set off with black cummerbunds and red tarbooshes.

After we were joined by the R.M. he and I immediately recognised each other's accent. A ship from England was great but somebody straight from Ireland was big stuff. He was hungry for news because, as he explained, the last aerogramme from two elderly aunts living in the small town of Bray near the Sugar Loaf mountain, just south of Dublin, had taken three months in transit. To his dismay, practically all of the precious space had been taken up with the news that their old cocker spaniel had developed cancer and had been put down by a very nice young vet. I asked if they lived on Killarney Road. Correct! I could hardly believe it; nor could he when I explained that I was that vet, though not a particularly nice one. I had attended the home of these two ladies during the time of my locum for Trevor Scott in Bray. I distinctly remembered having seen a photograph on their mantlepiece showing my new-found friend, Judge Greene, standing in tropical gear on the running board of a box-body station wagon with coconut palms in the background.

More happened in a single day in Zanzibar than might have taken place in Beira in a month of Sundays. The days passed pleasantly between lolling on the ship watching the activity in the harbour and exploring the island. I had always had a great ambition to own a white beachcomber's suit. Ironically, the day before we sailed I was a sitting duck for an Indian tailor who rolled out a few yards of white cotton drill as I passed and enthusiastically volunteered to make me one on the spot. I immediately retraced my steps when he shouted after me, 'Special price Bwana, only one pound'. The fact that I was sailing next morning presented no problem for the self-confident enthusiast so it was arranged that I would call back that evening before boarding for the last time. When I called on my way to the ship I was disappointed that the deadline had not been met, even though an assistant had been recruited to work on the trousers while the Master Tailor guided the lapels of the jacket through the Singer sewing machine. The tailor said 'No problem'; he would deliver it personally to the ship, but the pound had to be paid up front. On the following morning the hatches had been battened down and most of the little boats were making their way back to the shore. As I stood at the rail to say farewell to Zanzibar and my pound I spotted a rowing boat being paddled out furiously towards the ship. Sure enough, there was the figure of the conscientious tailor seated upright in the stern urging his crew on. As he drew in on the ship he stood up, unconcerned about the danger to himself in the wobbling craft, and threw a paper package with an almighty heave high into the air. It landed with a thud near my feet. Soon after my grateful thanks of '*assante sana*' to the tailor, the siren blew and we moved off. Although I was itching to try on my suit, it took me some time to detach myself from the beauty of the scene as the low sky-line, fringed with coconut palms gradually receded in the glare of the early morning sun.

Below in the cabin my beachcomber's suit fitted me like a glove. Later, after a day or two in Dar es Salaam it had to be handed over to the hotel *dhobi* (washerman) for washing. That was the advantage of cotton drill - it could be washed. Next day it came back beautifully ironed but, sadly, the trousers ended well above the ankles and the jacket could not be buttoned without a deep intake of breath. Alas, the cotton had not been pre-shrunk! However, the expenditure of a pound had provided great entertainment, and the tailor was happy, as was the dhobi who acquired a well-fitting suit.

I did not visit Zanzibar again until 1982, thirty-seven years later. A few days before my departure for my first return visit I happened to attend a wedding at which my friend Trevor Scott was also a guest. While he and I chatted together outside the church, my friend suggested that I might like to meet a couple of his clients who had spent many years in Africa. I was intrigued when they were introduced as Judge and Mrs Greene and then dumbfounded as it unfolded that, yes indeed, they were the Greenes who had entertained me and my friends in Zanzibar so many years ago. They were long retired and for many years had been living on the foothills of the Sugar Loaf Mountain; during the previous twenty-two years I myself had been living two miles east of that mountain, which was the last bit of Ireland I had seen in November 1944 after the convoy sailed from Liverpool!

The Greene's had kept in touch with Zanzibar through the Court Interpreter, a dignified Arab called Hassan, who had visited them in Ireland. During his stay he had developed a taste for a particular brand of Irish cheese called 'Galtee'. At that time the economies of Zanzibar and Tanganyika, by then both federated under the name of Tanzania, were desperately short of hard currency and there were practically no foreign consumer goods in the shops. On the eve of my departure for Zanzibar Mrs Greene called with a food parcel containing a generous lump of Galtee cheese for their friend. Two days later - mark you, not ten weeks as in 1944 - I was in Zanzibar where I made my way, with the food parcel, along a narrow street to Hassan's house. The meeting was delightful and marked the beginning of a warm friendship that lasted until his death some five years later. During this period I visited Zanzibar and the Island of Pemba annually as Technical Consultant to a livestock improvement project financed by the Irish Department of Foreign Affairs.

At the time of our first meeting Hassan was already an elderly gentleman enjoying the company of his many neighbours of long standing. On each of my visits his granddaughters popped in to greet him and to curtsy gracefully and shake hands with the visitor from Ireland. His memory went back a long way and on subsequent visits he entertained me to fascinating stories of his own experiences from the turn of the century onwards. These were supplemented by others handed down by his father who, as a petty officer in the Royal Navy, had been engaged in patrolling the Indian Ocean in search of slave ships, following the abolition of the slave trade.

Zanzibar had lost much of its exotic romance between my first visit in 1944 and the eighties. There was political turmoil and violence during the late fifties and early sixties followed by a mutiny of the police in 1964. The Sultan was deposed and a republic was established which aligned itself with China and Eastern Europe. The narrow, twisting streets in the ancient town, which had been there long before Livingstone prepared his last expedition to the mainland in 1866 in his search for the Nile, were tatty; most of the beautiful carved doors were gone and there was practically nothing in the shops. Worse still, high-rise concrete apartment blocks covered acres and acres of land on the edge of the old town.

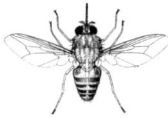

CHAPTER SIX

Dar Es Salaam to Mpwapwa

Dar es Salaam of yesteryear. Three humid nights on the veranda of an over-crowded hotel. Colourful, multiracial clamour at the Railway Station as passengers depart for destinations along the 700 mile journey up-country, following the route taken by Stanley seventy years previously. The awe-inspiring beauty of the mountainous country at Morogoro. Arrival at Gulwe after midnight, 250 miles from Dar, and onwards by dirt track to Mpwapwa.

The sun had reached its zenith and was casting short shadows on the deck by the time we entered the landlocked harbour of Dar es Salaam, so aptly named the 'Haven of Peace'. Even the rusted hulk of the German battleship, scuppered in 1916, and now half-submerged in the unruffled turquoise water did nothing to disturb the tranquillity of the scene.

Once again, policemen and officials from Immigration, Customs and Health swarmed on board and set up their desks in the ship's dining room which had been cleared for the purpose. As a Government official, I was excused the formality of proving that my financial affairs were in order and having to pay a deposit of fifty pounds to cover the cost of my repatriation, if that became necessary! I was then whisked off to the New Africa Hotel which I was correctly informed was the best hotel in Dar es Salaam. When I subsequently saw the others, including the Splendid Hotel, I learnt how misleading the adjective 'best' can be.

In those days the New Africa was a two storied building with an attractive red tiled roof. It was full to the gunnels so I was allocated an antiquated iron bed on an upstairs veranda partly screened off from the next bed by a rickety old wardrobe. This decorous concession seemed superfluous when I peeped round the improvised screen and saw one of my cabin mates, with whom I had travelled all the way from Liverpool, lying on the bed, stripped to the waist to get the benefit of any little breeze that was going. My bed was draped with a tired off-white mosquito net that smelt of the coconut oil from which the local soap was made, though it did not seem to have had much contact with soap for some time. It was the first mosquito net I had seen since I purchased my own away back at Griffiths McAlister in London. It was an exciting reminder that here I was actually starting life in the tropics where, as I was soon to learn, a sound mosquito net was far more comforting than a soft mattress.

Next day I was collected at the hotel by Sandy Milne, the Provincial Veterinary Officer for Eastern Province. He was a Scot and although he had qualified from Edinburgh only a few years previously he was already in charge of a whole province. Judging by his sallow complexion, which contrasted with his jet black hair, he had been in Dar es Salaam for some time and obviously knew his way around. He took me under his wing and I soon warmed to him and began to enjoy his laid-back attitude to the minor frustrations of Dar and the way he took them in his stride with his pawky sense of humour. He told me that I would be leaving by train for the Veterinary Headquarters at Mpwapwa on the following Tuesday. That left much to be done in two working days. Top priority was given to the signing of the Governor's Visitors' Book at Government House. The Governor was the supremo for the whole of Tanganyika and protocol was strict in those days. Next job was to report my arrival to the Secretariat. They sent me on to the Treasury where I learnt, to my delight, that I had been on half-pay for the past six months. I was not only delighted, I was greatly relieved because by then I was nearly stony-broke.

I was now able to open a bank account, buy provisions for 'up country' and engage house servants. Sandy's cook sent the word around and by Monday, on the eve of my departure for Mpwapwa, there were several candidates waiting at the Veterinary Office armed with their precious testimonials which were passports to the coveted world of employment in the households of Wazungus (Europeans). The interviews were conducted in Kiswahili by Sandy, who also scrutinised the testimonials a few of which were liable to be coded. For example, 'Juma has a rather taking personality . . .' meaning 'keep store cupboard locked'. 'A relaxed personality' was the signal for 'bone idle'.

After the shortlisting by Sandy final decisions, which could have important consequences for all of us, had to be made with due care. I fancied Huseni, henceforth to be known as *Mpishi*, the Kiswahili for cook. He was a mature, rather austere, dignified Muslim smartly attired in sparkling white trousers with knife-edged creases and a white shirt topped-off by a red fez on his head. Around forty, some seventeen years older than me, he subsequently tended to treat me in a slightly patronising manner and frowned on schoolboyish exuberance. In contrast, Selemani, a candidate for the post of 'House Boy', was a shy, droopy fellow dressed in a crumpled off-white *kanzu* that reached from head to foot and, being a Muslim, he wore a soft white cap precariously balanced on the back of his head as if it were going to fall off at any minute. He was about my own age and much less self-assured than *Mpishi*. But there was something about him and, almost against my better judgement, I offered him the job. It was a great decision. He turned out to be a con-firmed cynic with well-developed pragmatism and an unfailing dry sense of humour. Incidentally, his hat never did fall off during the next two years! He treated me with the prescribed degree of respect but seemed to do so with his tongue in his cheek, especially when pulling my leg. We developed a veiled camaraderie largely based, I always suspected, on a mutual fear of offending *Mpishi*'s sense of decorum.

They were an admirable pair. They spoke no English and at that stage my Kiswahili was rudimentary, so Sandy explained to *Mpishi* that I was going 'up-country' the very next morning, two hundred and fifty miles away in bush, and would probably spend a lot of time on safari anywhere in Tanganyika. Although they were both from the Coast and would each be leaving their wife behind, this presented no problem. Having secured the jobs, their sole concern was to negotiate a monstrous advance of salary. After a prolonged discussion in Swahili Sandy advised me that they had both returned to the real world and informed me of the agreed sum. Thereupon, impressive handshakes were exchanged. These involved the grasping of the four fingers of one of the party's right hand between the fingers and thumb of the other's. The erect thumb of the person receiving the hand shake was then grasped tightly by the other. The process was immediately repeated by the person who had received the first handshake. It was indeed impressive. The deal was done!

They were both waiting outside the railway station the following afternoon when I arrived with my loads on the ancient solid-tyred Albion lorry that the Veterinary Office had provided. *Mpishi* immediately took over, summoned porters and supervised the transfer of the loads to the luggage van. It was a little embarrassing to compare my pile of boxes with their luggage which consisted of a bag or box of private possessions and a sleeping roll for each.

I can still see the congestion and hear the clamour on the platform as more and more passengers and their friends - Europeans, Indians and Africans - kept arriving. European families dressed in safari jackets, still with their sun helmets on, stood in groups here and there along the platform chatting with their friends while *ayahs* (nurses) kept a watchful eye on the children. Porters pushed their trolleys through the noisy crowd. Eventually doors began to bang, last minute packages were stuffed through the windows, the whistle blew, final greetings were shouted and with a great puff of steam from the engine we were on our way.

With my Cambridge studies on the exploration of tropical Africa fresh in mind it was fascinating to remind myself that I was now following almost precisely the same route to Mpwapwa that Stanley had taken seventy-four years previously during his expedition to Lake Tanganyika in his search for Dr Livingstone. One difference was that he had started from Bagamoyo about forty miles north of where Dar es Salaam now stands. It was by no means the only difference. Stanley had taken fifty-seven days to reach Mpwapwa with his caravan of *wapagazi* (porters) and donkeys while I was to cover the same distance of approximately 250 miles in fourteen hours and in much greater comfort.

Given the state of development of the country the Tanganyika Railways were impressive. The coaches were made of timber and in accordance with the universal custom of the time they were designated First, Second and Third Class. (See illust.) Being a Government Official I had the privilege of occupying a small compartment all to myself in a First Class carriage and, in due course, I made my way down the corridor to the dining car. Everything was spotless. A friendly group invited me to join them for a glass of beer. I learnt that the construction of the first stretch of the Central Railway line on which we were travelling had been started by the Germans in 1905, with the aid of Greeks whom they had

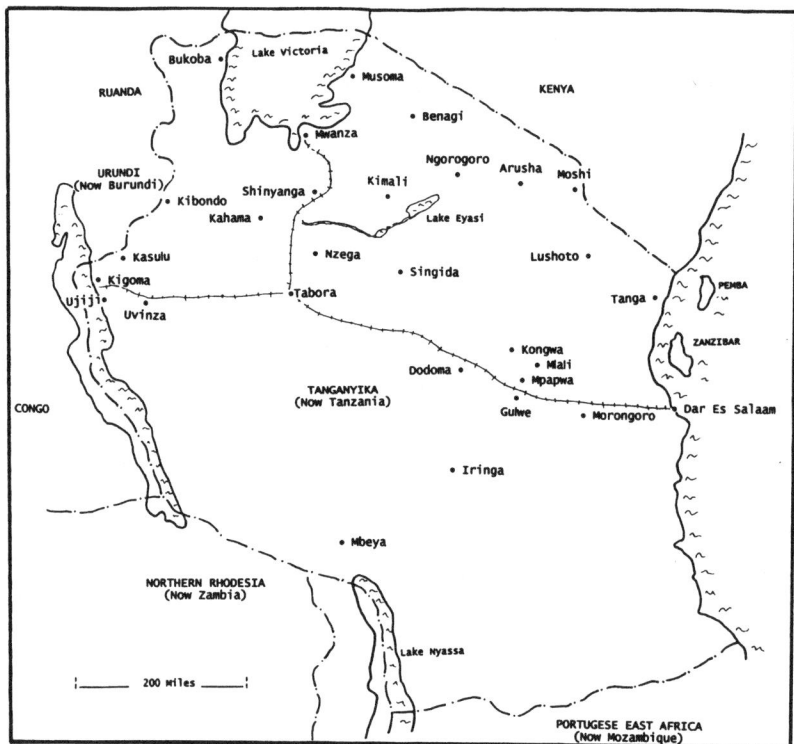

Diagrammatic map showing the relative locations of places mentioned in the text.

brought in for the purpose. It reached Morogoro in 1907 and entered Tabora, almost 500 miles from the coast, in 1912 and finally reached Kigoma on Lake Tanganyika in 1914. At Kigoma a steamship, the *Liemba*, belonging to the Railway Administration provided a regular passenger and cargo service down the lake to Northern Rhodesia (now Zambia). A great deal had happened since Stanley met Dr Livingstone seventy-three years previously at Ujiji, a small village some ten miles south of Kigoma. A branch line from Tabora to Mwanza on the shores of Lake Victoria had been built by the British in 1921. From there sizeable steamers extended the service to Uganda and Kenya and to other centres in Tanganyika on both sides of the lake. A year later, when I subsequently travelled by train to Kigoma and saw, with my own eyes, the Belgian Congo on the far distant horizon across Lake Tanganyika it was brought home to me how much had been done to open up Central Africa in such a short space of time. For example, by 1914 it took only some fifty-seven hours to travel the 778 miles from Dar es Salaam to Kigoma by rail compared with between four and six months by foot caravan.

The railway network, including a line running east to west from Tanga on the coast to Arusha in Northern Tanganyika, played a vital role in communications because of the poor road structure within the country. All the roads, apart from some fifty miles of tarmacadam, within this vast territory of 364,881 square miles - more than eleven times the size of the whole of Ireland - were bare earth and as such were frequently impassable during the rains. Most of the telephone lines ran along the railway so it was not surprising that the administrative headquarters of many of the Provinces and Districts were situated on the railway. I was particularly interested in my companions' account of the railways because I was already aware that the Central Line was of great significance to the work of the Veterinary Department in controlling the spread of rinderpest, the dreaded disease of cattle which was to occupy much of my time during the next three years.

An amusing story told during this, my first 20 mph sundowner, illustrated the privileged, easy-going life that was enjoyed by the Europeans of those days. There was only one dentist in the whole of Tanganyika and as he was stationed in Dar es Salaam government officers were obliged to make the journey to him when necessary. On one occasion a well-known character who was returning from Dar with his first set of dentures had spent the morning drinking in the dining car. He had to run out in the middle of lunch to the toilet where the upper set of his dentures shot down the pan during the last retch. He was sufficiently sober to pull the communication cord - after all, it was an emergency! The train screeched along the rails on locked wheels, then jolted to a halt. No doubt, this was accompanied by the discharging of volleys of coconuts, pineapples, bananas and yams from the overhead racks in the Third Class carriages. The toothless passenger called on his pals in speech even more slurred than before to accompany him down the line in search of a soiled patch between the rails. There was the denture glinting in the sunshine surrounded by the splattered remains of a lunch. The Indian Guard was as delighted as the rest of the party and there was no further enquiry, no penalty for improper use - it was indeed an emergency, there being no other dentist in the whole of the country.

After sunset we were leaving the coastal plain, still less than a thousand feet above sea level, and beginning the climb towards Mororgoro which was a major road junction and administrative centre. The town lies at the foot of the Ulugura Mountains which rise to a height of some 8,000 feet and stretch along the side of the railway for several miles. As the train laboured up the long incline to Mororgoro I stood in awe on the veranda staring at the massive mountain range bathed in the silvery light of a full moon in a cloudless sky. I was deeply moved by the beauty and sheer size of the scene and in my reverie I fell deeply in love with Tanganyika and felt so grateful that the fateful decision made six months ago in the Colonial Office, now so far away in time and space, had brought me here.

Later on, after an excellent dinner I returned to my cabin to find the bed made up with crisp white sheets under the comforting protection of a mosquito net. I slept fitfully as the train toiled its way higher and higher through the cool mountain air towards Gulwe station where we arrived at 2.30 a.m. This was the wayside station for Mpwapwa, now only twelve miles away. As the only white man descending from the train I was easily recognised by the driver of the veterinary lorry who had been sent to meet me. A number of swinging hurricane lamps converged on us as we made our way to the guard's van. They transpired to be held by an abundance of porters eager to assist us in loading the boxes on to the lorry.

The journey to Mpwapwa was a fitting introduction to road travel up country. The dirt road had not been 'made up' since the recent short rains so the pace was slow as we bumped over the uneven surface. At some of the many culverts storm water had cut deep channels over which we had to crawl at a snail's pace. Like most vehicles in Tanganyika during the war the lorry had seen better times. The shock absorbers, such as they were, seemed to be synchronised with the headlamps which kept flickering out at the heaviest bumps and had to be thumped by the turney boy (the driver's assistant) to get them on again. There were no huts or other signs of human habitation at the roadside as we drove through the dense thorn bush until our lights picked up the thatched mud huts and small houses of Mpwapwa village, where Stanley had camped seventy-four years before.

The village stands on the plain at the mouth of a river gorge that opens out after a mile into an extensive area of relatively flat land, known as Kikombo, tucked away in the Ukaguru Mountains. The little stream that bubbles through the narrow defile endows the valley with a cool, moist climate quite different from that of the semi-arid plain across which we had driven from Gulwe. The lushness of the vegetation, picked up in the headlights, provided a reassuring welcome to the large valley of Kikombo that accommodated the headquarters, laboratories and experimental farms of the Veterinary Department.

At the end of the gorge we passed the headquarters building to the right and splashed through a ford into the open terrain of Kikombo. Half a mile further on I was deposited at a small rest house and almost immediately a figure carrying a hurricane lantern appeared on the veranda and exclaimed, '*Jambo* Rob, *karibu sana*' (hello Rob, hearty welcome). It was the unmistakable voice of my old friend Mac who had arrived six weeks ahead of me. The arrival of trains at Gulwe was unpredictable so he had slept fitfully with one ear cocked. *Mpishi* and Selemani had travelled reasonably well on the back of the lorry despite the unaccustomed cold air. They were greeted warmly by Mac's servants who emerged from the darkness and joined in the unloading of the lorry before escorting them to their own quarters. Mac was quite unchanged and even in the dimly lit environment of the rest house was even more enthusiastic about all that Mpwapwa had to offer than he had been about his activities at Cambridge. It was a wonderful reunion and after several cups of tea it was 5 a.m. Sleep was out of the question.

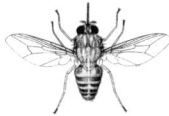

CHAPTER SEVEN

Mpwapwa:
A Veterinary Enclave

Headquarters and laboratories of the Veterinary Department located in an idyllic mountainous setting from which the veterinary needs of a territory thirteen times the size of Ireland were served by a skeleton staff of expatriates supported by a highly effective cadre of African personnel throughout the length and breath of the country.

T he village of Mpwapwa was, and still is, the headquarters of the Mpwapwa District. Nevertheless the veterinary enclave, tucked into the Ukaguru Mountains at the head of the narrow valley about a mile from the actual village, was known throughout Tanganyika as Mpwapwa because it was the administrative headquarters of the Department of Veterinary Science and Animal Husbandry. It also accommodated the Department's veterinary laboratory and experimental farms. The enclave consisted of a network of wide valleys covering an area of some 4,000 acres, though the Department probably 'owned' two other largely uninhabited adjoining valleys and hills as the station eventually extended to 17,000 acres. Most of the buildings and residences were located in Kikombo, the first valley one encounters driving in from the village, just beyond a gently rolling nine hole golf course set against the spectacular backdrop of Kiboriani Mountain which rises to 7,500 feet. (See illust.)

The natural vegetation consisted of deciduous thicket, much of which had been cleared, giving wide expanses of grassland. Lying at an altitude of almost 3,700 feet, the climate was reasonably cool, the only really hot month being November when temperatures normally rose

54

above 90' F degrees just before the rains. The rains, though extremely variable in distribution and amount from year to year, generally fell between December and April with quite a dry spell normally in February. In general it was a most pleasant oasis compared with the dreary thorn bush of the surrounding semi-arid plains of Central Tanganyika.

During my first few days Mac introduced me with characteristic enthusiasm to the Tanganyika Veterinary Services in general and to Mpwapwa in particular. The Director of Veterinary Services H. J. Lowe, who had impressed me greatly by entertaining me to lunch at the Shelbourne Hotel in Dublin six months previously, and the Acting Chief Veterinary Research Officer, Jack Wilde, had both recently left for Nairobi to attend an inter-territorial conference. In their absence a Senior Veterinary Officer, Willie Burns, who had joined the Department in 1923, was in charge of the veterinary affairs throughout the whole country and such was the shortage of staff that young Mac was in charge of the laboratory services. For my first night he had invited Willie and his attractive young wife, Elsa, to dinner. During the conversation it was exciting to find oneself being drawn back into the fascinating history of the extraordinary country.

Much more was revealed at the relaxed sessions at Headquarters next morning with another Senior Veterinary Officer, Neil Reid, and the Chief Clerk, Ray Rainer, the other two European members of the staff. I learnt that the entire graduate veterinary staff of the country had been reduced from twenty-seven at the beginning of the war to nineteen. Several of the veterinary officers were, of course, on long leave (generally in South Africa during the war) at any one time. There was also one African Assistant Veterinary Officer, Godfrey Mhina, who had recently completed his training at Makerere College in Uganda, an institution affiliated with the University of London. The veterinary staff was supplemented by an establishment of twenty-nine European livestock officers and stock inspectors, a pasture research officer and a chemist, but seven of these posts including the latter two were vacant.

The provision of veterinary and animal husbandry services for Tanganyika's six million cattle, five million sheep and goats and a hundred thousand donkeys, scattered over 364,000 square miles, was a daunting task for such a small professional staff. To put these figures into some kind of perspective it is worth noting that the Republic of Ireland which is about thirteen times smaller than Tanganyika had at that time 420 registered veterinarians for only four million cattle and two and a half million sheep.

Fortunately, the Department was blessed with twenty four African Veterinary Assistants and several Animal Husbandry Assistants all of whom had been trained at Mpwapwa. They were greatly valued as key men in provincial and district offices and at the laboratory. In addition, there were about 300 Veterinary Guards stationed throughout the length and breadth of the country without whom, as I subsequently learnt, the Department could not have survived. Each provincial and district office had its own complement and many were stationed on their own in small towns and bigger villages. In my subsequent experience I found them to be responsible, practical men, highly competent at basic clinical procedures such as inoculations, blood sampling, castrations and wound dressing. They also had basic knowledge of meat inspection and hygiene, they supervised and gave instruction in hide and skin drying, conducted the livestock census and collected information about outbreaks of disease and other matters. In short, they were the Department's front men in the field and, above all, its eyes and ears especially in the more remote parts of the country. They were proud of their vocation and their uniform. The latter consisted of a khaki tunic and shorts, a handsome leather belt with a well-shone brass buckle, embossed unfairly with the ambiguous letters "VD", blue puttees and a blue fez. Always spotlessly turned out they drew themselves to attention on meeting a more senior member of the Department and saluted with a firm stamp of the right foot, followed by a forthright "*Jambo Bwana*" – seemingly a legacy passed down from the days before German East Africa passed to British Administration under the League of Nations mandate.

In due course, I became aware of the extraordinary range of activities in which the Department was involved. Its primary responsibility was, of course, the control and prevention of disease in large populations on a herd and flock basis rather than the treatment of individual animals. This was dictated by the low cash value of individual animals. For example, in those days the price of a bullock was about two pounds. Moreover, the infrastructure of the country except for a few localities was completely inadequate for attending to individual animals. The highest priority was given to rinderpest, or cattle plague, because of its appalling mortality rate as well as Tanganyika's position on the route along which the disease had swept on its way to the Rhodesias and South Africa at the turn of the century. Next in importance came trypanosomiasis, the equivalent in animals of sleeping sickness in humans, which is transmitted by the tsetse fly. This disease rendered vast areas of the country uninhabitable for man and animals. Consequently, heavy concentrations of cattle, sheep and goats were confined to range land which became so over grazed during the dry season that soil erosion was common. Such erosion, in turn, further reduced the carrying capacity of the tsetse-free areas. East Coast fever, which is transmitted by ticks, was prevalent in certain areas where the climate was suitable for the tick vector. In such areas calf mortality was usually about 50 per cent with the result that the incremental rate of the cattle population was so depressed that the affected range was characterised by an abundance of grass and a scarcity of cattle. Other serious diseases included contagious bovine pleuropneumonia, anthrax, blackquarter, brucellosis, foot and mouth disease, heartwater, tropical redwater, tuberculosis, rabies and a wide variety of debilitating, potentially fatal conditions caused by a variety of helminth infestations.

The Department had always taken an holistic approach to animal health, its philosophy being that disease was inseparable from nutrition and husbandry. Therefore, it was deeply involved in water and soil conservation, the establishment of grazing reserves for the dry season, and genetic improvement of the indigenous breeds of livestock. It was also responsible for the development and control of the livestock industry. Provincial Veterinary Officers fixed prices and allocated quotas to cattle dealers in such a way that destocking of seriously over-stocked areas was encouraged. The Department developed and supervised stock routes along which trade cattle were trekked to a meat factory operated by Messrs Liebigs many miles away in Kenya and to other consuming centres. Here and there the routes had to go through tracts of land where the tsetse fly, trypanosomiasis and other serious diseases, such as East Coast fever, were endemic. Other responsibilities included meat hygiene at the larger centres, control and improvement of the hide and skin industry and the improvement of clarified butter and ghee production in areas where there was a surplus of fresh milk. In short, the Department was responsible for all matters relating directly to domesticated livestock; all in all a very extensive and logical remit. The Department of Agriculture concerned itself almost exclusively with the cultivation and marketing of arable crops.

Mac, who was temporarily in charge of the Laboratory, took me around the rest of Mpwapwa and what I saw during the next few days transmitted his enthusiasm to me in full measure. Our first stop was the laboratory complex situated near the foot of Kiborani Mountain just beyond the golf course and most of the residences. The actual laboratories were housed in a single storey building built by the Germans around 1905. A cool veranda running along the front of the building connected the adjoining labs. The building also housed an electrical generator and a most effective Heath Robinson gas generator, based on the principle of the Primus stove, that converted paraffin into gas for the autoclaves and the Bunsen burners. The actual laboratory equipment, though simple, provided the essentials for microscopy, bacteriology, the elementary virology of the time and chemistry. Despite its simplicity the Laboratory was capable of diagnosing most of the important diseases of livestock occurring in the country and producing certain vaccines.

Clustered around the main building there was a library; stores; a post-mortem room; a laboratory animal unit; *boma*s or kraals with eight to ten foot high walls for the overnight protection of cattle, sheep and goats against lions and leopards; an infectious diseases isolation unit known as 'the Rinderpest Hospital'; and a small zoo for the study of the transmission of disease between wildlife and domestic animals. Apparently, the most substantial of the cattle *boma*s, a particularly large one with stone-built walls, had been used during the First World War to house prisoners of war. Nearby there was a cattle dipping tank, used for the control of tick-borne diseases. Further afield there were two experimental dairy farms, another cattle dip, a poultry farm and a brick works. This particular dip (at Nunge Dairy) was built by the Germans. At the time of writing it is still in use and is reputed to be the first-ever dip built in East Africa. The whole complex was an impressive tribute to those pioneers who over the years had created these valuable facilities in this remote valley in the face of logistical difficulties.

Mac was likely to be transferred to a field station at any time and it seemed that I would remain at Mpwapwa to assist the hard-pressed

Acting Chief Research Officer. It was hard to conceal my amazement and excitement as Mac showed me more and more. At long last, after eighteen months of seemingly irrelevant postgraduate studies, picking at little bits of veterinary work, interminable waiting and travel, I was about to start practising my chosen profession fulltime with all these wonderful facilities at my disposal. Little did I realise how soon I was going to be thrown into the deep end with sole responsibility for keeping the whole shebang afloat for almost a year.

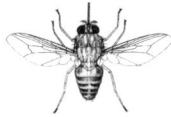

CHAPTER EIGHT

Settling In

Sharing a Rest House and a double complement of staff with Mac, an old friend from Cambridge - two cooks, a fridge operated by paraffin oil, candlelight dinners and gramaphone music. At long last into real veterinary work; vaccine production and diagnostic procedures at the lab and exciting clinical cases including the sudden death of an antelope in the Zoo caused by anthrax.

Mac and I were to share the rest house until either he or I were transferred to the field. It was a modest tin-roofed house with two bedrooms, a bathroom, dining room, sitting room and a 'mosquito-proof' veranda that had seen better times. The kitchen was at the end of the garden beside the servants' quarters. Wonderful work was done in that kitchen on the wood-burning Dover stove that belched smoke because the firebox door was invariably left open to accommodate hefty lengths of firewood. To have cut them to size would have been considered unnecessary hard work.

We now had a combined staff and never quite knew how they all fitted into the servants' quarters. In Africa job demarcation was unshakeable so between us we now had two cooks, two 'house boys' and one cook's boy/gardener. The latter was the dogsbody who did most of the hard work, such as gathering firewood, peeling potatoes, scrubbing pots, lighting tilly lamps and operating the contraption for the evening baths. The contraption was a 44-gallon drum mounted at a height of some six feet on two supporting walls outside the bathroom. There was a fireplace immediately below the drum and the latter was plumbed through the bathroom wall to the hot tap. The unfortunate garden boy was berated unmercifully in a self-righteous manner by the rest of the staff on the occasions when he was not back from the village in good time to light the fire and have the Bwanas' bath water at the right temperature by sundown.

My *Mpishi* was delighted by the variety of locally produced raw materials with which to practise his trade. Obviously, he had not read Henry Morton Stanley's book *How I found Livingstone*. When Stanley met Sheik Thani, with the latter's huge caravan "encamped under the grateful umbrage of a huge Mtamba sycamore" at Mpwapwa village on a second journey in 1874, the Sheik advised him emphatically to "stop here for two or three days, give your tired animals some rest; collect all the *pagazis* [*wapagazi*, Swahili for 'porters'] you can, fill your insides with fresh milk, sweet potatoes, beef, mutton, ghee, honey, beans, *matama*, *maweri* and nuts ..." *Mpishi* soon found that he could add chickens, butter and cream to the Sheik's list, as well as pork, bacon and ham from Bwana Bain's bacon factory 50 miles away beyond the mountains.

Work at the Lab started at 7 a.m. and finished officially at 4 p.m. with an hour for breakfast and lunch at 8 a.m. and 1 p.m. respectively. That left barely three hours for recreation before sunset. There was much to do including shooting, tennis, golf and swimming; the latter in a concrete pool officially called the irrigation tank to conceal the irresponsible expenditure of public money. The laboratory also had three riding horses and a remarkably sure-footed mule. After the afternoon's recreation one generally repaired with the companions of the day to somebody's house for a sundowner which usually consisted of a cold beer. That took care of the ration of four dozen bottles of beer and one of whisky per person that arrived once a month from Dar. Consequently, chronic alcoholism was never a problem at Mpwapwa but the acute form of the condition was sometimes seen during stress-related blow-outs, involving the whole European population, that occasionally occurred spontaneously shortly after the arrival of the ration.

The normal sundowner was an excellent switch-off. It punctuated the end of the day's activities and prepared one for a relaxing bath, dinner and a quiet read before bed. There was nowhere else to go after dark other than to have dinner with friends. Anyway one did not wander far away on foot at night for fear of lions and leopards. Our evening meal in the rest house gradually took on a character of its own. Having two groups of staffs, one team could alternate with the other. This added variety to the four-course menu; as well, my cook's patronising manner introduced a competitive element that progressively improved the quality.

Selemani had fallen in love with my portable gramophone and the eight records that had survived the journey. He took it upon himself to work through the records, winding the handle between courses and changing the needles when necessary. Before long Mac and I and, indeed, the entire household were addicted to 'Lily Marlene', 'Moonlight in Mayo', selections of Gilbert and Sullivan and a few excerpts of more serious music. Selemani never missed a chance and I can still recite the verses of his favourite, 'Underneath the lamplight at the barrack gate. . .' word for word. Sadly, before long, the irreplaceable needles were too blunt for further use and the dinners became more of a nutritional necessity than a celebration. We became more conscious of the chirping of the cicadas, the croaking of frogs and the occasional bark of a jackal. Then one night Selemani served the soup and drifted quietly, like a ghost in his long white kanzu, into the shadows where the gramophone stood idle. Suddenly, the room was filled with the gentle strains of 'Underneath the lamplight'. He had discovered that the sharp spike at the top of a sisal leaf did the trick. We were back in business, with an inexhaustible supply of needles just outside in the back garden!

There were other shortages too though the staples that were produced within the country, such as flour, rice, sugar, cooking oil, salt, soap etcetera, were invariably available in the little Indian *dukas* (shops) in the village. Imported goods, from gramophone needles to radios, refrigerators and motor cars were either unobtainable or in very short supply because of the war. Consequently, it was comforting during the unpacking of my own loads to find that practically all of the precious contents were intact after their long journey from another world.

Those who had been in the country for some years prized short wave radios powered by car batteries, refrigerators operated by paraffin oil and, of course, pre-war motor cars. Willie Burns, though he was Deputy Director of the Department, enjoyed even greater status from his ownership of a vintage Rolls Royce with an estate body made of local timber. It created an incongruous picture as the Rolls Royce emerged from a clump of flat-topped Acacia trees, followed by a cloud of dust on its daily journey from Willie's house to Head Office. In those early days, much of what I saw just didn't seem real: a Rolls Royce; a Head Office with a corrugated iron roof along which a colony of monkeys from the overhanging trees raced creating such a racket that discussions in the Director's office (often heated) were compliantly suspended mid-sentence; a zoo with high walls to keep lions and leopards out. Then there was the odd combination of laboratories, dairy farms, a nine-hole golf course of sorts, pull-and-let-go sanitation, hot baths, cold beer from fridges running on paraffin, bacon and eggs for breakfast and crème caramel with double cream for dinner. All this, and much more, in an oasis sitting in the middle of the dry thorn bush of Central Tanganyika, seventy miles from the nearest town, Dodoma, and the whole lot two to three months away from home by air mail, and old Mac from Cambridge thrown in for good measure. Unbelievable!

It was now time to settle into some real work as Mac's assistant at the laboratory. The laboratory complex was full of life with much coming and going, especially on the veranda of the main building (see illust.). The chemistry lab was located to the right at the end of the veranda under the shade of a large tree. In the absence of the Biochemist, on secondment to Kenya, it was used mainly for the analysis of samples of clarified butter and ghee from all parts of the country, and the preparation of laboratory reagents. The next two rooms served as offices for the Livestock Officer and two South African Apprentice Stock Inspectors. Further down the veranda were the offices for the Acting Chief Veterinary Research Officer, and Veterinary Research Officers, a 'clean lab' for microbiology, a large general lab for microscopy, histology and haematology. At the very end was a spacious area housing wash-up sinks with stainless steel benches, autoclaves, and other sterilisers. This large room was a busy place enlivened by the hiss of steam from the autoclaves, the clinking of glassware including crates of beer bottles - about which, more later - the clatter of buckets on the wet floor and the chatter of the inmates. It was, amongst other things, virtually a rinderpest vaccine factory.

The actual laboratory staff consisted of Mac, Godfrey the African Assistant Veterinary Officer, three Laboratory Technicians and several laboratory attendants. Godfrey and the Laboratory Technicians were highly responsible, experienced people; the laboratory could not have functioned without them. Apart from the Chief Clerk, a Goan, they were the only English-speaking personnel. The rest of the staff spoke Kiswahili which was the lingua franca of the country.

The Chief Clerk, the inimitable Mr Almeida, presided over the general office at the back of the building. There was an excellent filing system that enabled any document to be retrieved within minutes, provided the file had been returned to its proper place in its cabinet. For as long as anybody could remember, however, Mr Almeida never had time to put the files away. Instead, he strewed the floor with little piles of precariously balanced files. Surprisingly though, he knew the configuration on the floors just as well as a Masai herd boy who cannot count knows instinctively when even one animal is missing from the herd. He could produce any file at the drop of a hat; but what a nightmare it was for anyone else who needed to catch up on correspondence over the weekend!

Letters were, of course, our main means of communication. How formal they were in those days. Some of the more formal ones from Dar es Salaam began 'Sir, I have the honour to inform you. . .' and ended 'I have the honour to be, Sir, your obedient servant.' The first link in the chain of command with the outside world was a pair of uniformed messengers who sat patiently on the veranda for hours on end and shuttled leisurely between the laboratory and Head Office. There was also a telephone line through Head Office that dealt badly, if at all, with the spoken word but admirably with telegrams.

Mac, with two months experience under his belt, concentrated on vaccine production, supervising the diagnostic work, administration and indoctrinating me. All this was more than a full-time job so I tended to relieve him of the clinical work of which there was no shortage as we had some 2,000 head of cattle, sheep, goats and pigs in total, as well as three riding horses, a herd of donkeys, poultry, some small laboratory animals and a zoo.

My transport was an old Royal Enfield motorbike, with sweeping handlebars and a hand operated gearshift, which today would be much sought after as a vintage classic. What a joy it was to spin through the crisp, morning air along narrow tracks towards the more remote valleys. At that time of day the mountains stood out in sharp relief against a huge backdrop of blue sky studded with puffy white clouds. But unforgettable for their beauty were the tenuous wisps of cloud, pure white in the early morning sun, clinging to the contours of the mountains halfway between the lower slopes and the peaks. As the temperature rose the wisps evaporated before one's eyes.

The donkeys gave us more trouble than any other animal. Nobody seemed to know why we had them. They were probably a legacy from the days, only a few years previously, when walking safaris were the order of the day in many parts of the country. There were several competing stallions in the herd, consequently as successive jennies came on heat there was much braying, kicking, biting and lacerations. Blowflies almost immediately laid their eggs in the wounds which were soon suppurating and crawling with maggots. The horrible wounds were a graphic warning that surgical intervention involving the intact skin should never be inflicted on animals out-of-doors in the tropics. For this reason, the bloodless method, using Burdizzo forceps to crush the spermatic cord, was used for the hundreds of thousands of castrations of cattle, sheep, goats and donkeys that were then being performed annually by Veterinary Guards throughout Tanganyika. Needless to say, Mac and I with youthful enthusiasm used the same method to reduce the competition within the herd at Mpwapwa.

Not long after my arrival I ran into a very exciting case. A bushbuck in the Zoo died suddenly. In any case of sudden death, particularly in Africa, one must eliminate the possibility of anthrax before opening the carcass for post-mortem examination. The reason for doing so is that in most species sudden death from anthrax is associated with a septicaemia in which the organisms are teeming in the blood. As soon as the bacilli are exposed to air they sporulate and in this form are capable of surviving for many years in the soil, as well as in the hides, skins and wool of infected animals. Therefore, it is imperative that no blood be spilt until the possibility of anthrax has been eliminated.

The diagnosis is made by gently pricking an ear vein and smearing a drop of blood on a glass slide. This must be done with due care because the disease is highly infectious for man as well as animals. In man sudden death or an early septicaemia with generalised symptoms is relatively rare but if infected blood or spores make contact with the skin the infection is liable to enter the body through an abrasion. A very painful bright-red pimple appears which develops rapidly into a blackish-red vesicle known as a malignant pustule. More pustules and vesicles appear, the surrounding tissues disintegrate and extensive swelling occurs. At this point a fatal septicaemia is likely to occur, so one must be extremely cautious in handling infective material. In certain circumstances, such as during the handling of wool, spores may be inhaled resulting in an acute, rapidly fatal pneumonia known as wool-sorters' disease. Sadly, this knowledge has been exploited by incorporating cultures of these organisms in aerosols for use in germ warfare.

There is a very simple and rapid staining procedure for *Bacillus anthracis*, so one can have the slide under the microscope within ten minutes. However, care must be taken to differentiate the rod-like organisms from other similarly shaped non-pathogenic bacilli that may invade the bloodstream from the intestine after death. Mac and I were ninety-nine per cent sure it was anthrax but, after all, it was our first case outside the classroom so we felt we had to run a confirmatory test. Regretably, that involved injecting a guinea pig with a drop of blood from the bushbuck. A day or two later the unfortunate creature was dead. Having satisfied ourselves with the diagnosis the carcass of the bushbuck was removed from the zoo with care to ensure that no blood was spilt. It was then incinerated. In 1945 there was no effective treatment for anthrax; the use of sulphonamides and penicillin was only in the early experimental stages. Fortunately, we had good stocks of vaccine so all of our livestock had to be immunised.

Shortly, after the case of anthrax occurred the Director of Veterinary Services, Mr Lowe, and Jack Wilde, the Acting Chief Veterinary Research Officer, returned from Nairobi. To the consternation of Mac and myself Jack was immediately told that there was a passage for him on a ship bound for the United Kingdom. This was to be his first home leave, already long overdue. Two days later he had packed and was on his way to Gulwe Station en route to Dar es Salaam, 250 miles away.

On that particular day, a Sunday, more than half the European population of Mpwapwa made one of its periodic excursions to the nearby lake at Kimagai, some twelve miles away. The staff and wives of the Veterinary Department numbered sixteen; there were another four Europeans at Mpwapwa Village outside the valley, namely the District Officer and his wife, the Principal of the African Secondary School and his wife, and their children. There were only two or three cars belonging to those making the trip so a departmental lorry was borrowed to accommodate the bachelors and a few servants who were delighted to have the trip. The lorry party travelled in style on armchairs thrown on at the various houses. It was delightful lounging on the chairs, the balmy air inflating our shirts as we sped through the bone dry thorn bush followed by a billowing cloud of dust. The lake was nothing spectacular but there were no others to choose from. Its main attraction was that it provided an opportunity for some unsophisticated sailing and an excuse to grill steaks for lunch. The yachts were fragile, home-made craft consisting of a light timber frame supporting a skin of tarred canvas. They barely carried two but there was no danger of drowning because even during the rains the water was never deeper than three feet. When they capsized all one had to do was catch the prow and walk to the shore.

The railway line from Gulwe to Dar es Salaam ran along the south shore of the lake so, as the afternoon wore on, our little flotilla sailed across to send one of its passengers, a very happy Jack Wilde who had boarded the train at Gulwe, on his way. The train slowed at the sight of the little group of *Wazunzu* (Europeans) at the side of the track and came to a halt with a friendly greeting from the Indian driver. Jack stepped down for handshakes, or kisses and hugs as appropriate, while his fellow passengers stretched their heads out the windows to watch the party good-naturedly. Further down the line, others in the Third Class carriages took the opportunity to detrain for a comfort stop. Finally, with a puff of steam and a cheery toot-toot from the engine the last of the comforted stoppers emerged from the long grass and climbed aboard, as did Jack. Such was the unhurried, informality of rail travel in Tanganyika.

Back at Mpwapwa the veterinary clinician found that he himself needed a clinician and discovered there was a doctor in the house. For a day or two I had become aware of a tender spot under a toenail. As the pain increased I began to limp. Selemani enquired, '*Taabu gani*, Bwana?' (What's the trouble, Bwana?) When I explained we both examined the spot. It was now bigger, about the size of a small pea, much softer and an angry purple in colour. Selemani immediately diagnosed the trouble as a jigger and gave his prognosis. '*Si kitu*' (it's OK) He would fix it.

The jigger, *Tunga penetrans*, is a small flea, only about 1 mm long, whose eggs are found in sandy soil or on the dusty floors of houses. Each egg produces a larva that pupates in a cocoon. In due course, a mature flea emerges. After fertilisation the female penetrates the skin of a suitable host of which man and pigs seem to be the most common. In man the preferred site is the tender skin under the toenails. Once embedded, the female sucks blood and begins to produce great numbers of eggs which accumulate in her abdomen causing it to swell progressively. The pressure on the surrounding tissues of the host causes inflammation and ulceration at the site, accompanied by intense pain. Eventually, she bursts and the eggs are expelled into the environment.

Originally the jigger was confined to tropical America but reputedly made its way across the Atlantic Ocean to West Africa early in the 1870s in ballast sand. From there the fleas spread rapidly to almost all parts of Africa and within 20 years they had reached the east coast. The rate at which this nasty little creature travelled from coast to coast is an interesting reminder of the extent to which direct contact existed between the indigenous people of the western, central and eastern zones of tropical Africa during the nineteenth century, even before the 'Dark Continent' was opened up by Europeans. A case in point concerns an African called Msiri, from the copper-rich region of Katanga to the south west of Lake Tanganyika, who started life as a porter and soon became a caravan leader. He brought in guns from Bagamoyo, some thousand miles away on the east coast of Tanganyika, for his own private army. By the time Stanley made his journey in 1871 from Bagamoyo to Ujiji on Lake Tanganyika in his search for Livingstone, Msiri was a powerful trader with caravans plying between the Atlantic port of Benguela (now Lobito) in Angola and Bagamoyo on the Indian Ocean, carrying such goods as copper, ivory, rubber, wax and, of course, slaves. The distance from coast to coast, via Katanga, was some two thousand miles. As successive generations of female jiggers completed their life cycles in the infested toes of caravan porters and released their eggs onto the dusty floors of huts at rest camps along the trade routes it would not take many years for the entire route to become infested with their eggs.

Of course, Selemani was not aware of all the details of this life cycle but he proved to be a master with a darning needle. I dutifully rested my foot on his knee. Thereupon, he gently enlarged the cavity, in which the rotund flea was lodged, by patiently teasing out the surrounding tissue until he was satisfied that he could remove the soft mass intact. This was important because the escape of eggs into the tissues is liable to produce a suppurating wound which can, in extreme cases, result in loss of a toe or worse. The disfigured toes of so many barefooted Africans was an indication of the widespread prevalence of this parasite.

Selemani was as delighted as I was by the successful removal of the jigger. For me the relief was bliss after the sting from a dab of iodine had worn off. He solemnly warned me not to walk around dusty rest houses in bare feet. *Mpishi* underlined the advice with a pious interjection, '*Ndeo, kweli sana*, Bwana' – (Yes, very true, Bwana). The bonding of our little family had progressed apace!

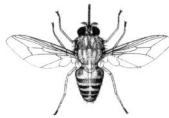

CHAPTER NINE

Flying Solo

Mac's sudden transfer to the field leaves the author in sole charge for the next ten months. Almost immediately a dog's brain is received for the diagnosis of rabies. Thereafter, high priority is given to satisfying insatiable demands for rinderpest vaccine to prevent the dread disease spreading southwards from Tanganyika as it had done fifty years previously.

A month after my arrival in Mpwapwa an outbreak of rinderpest occurred in Singida District, not far north of the strategically important Central Railway line. The news was disturbing; Head Office was tense. Mac was immediately posted to Singida. Two days later he was on his way and I was put in sole charge of the laboratory.

As so often happens at crucial moments, a most unwelcome distraction occurred just as I took over. The brain of a dog suspected of having suffered from rabies arrived from a remote part of the country. Half of the brain was preserved in formalin for histological examination; the other half was sealed in a jar of glycerine to preserve the virus in case transmission experiments had to be done. Both specimens were packed in a four gallon petrol can, known as a *debe*. The lid had been securely soldered in place to ensure that no leakage occurred in transit. To make assurance doubly sure, the *debe* was enclosed in a stout wooden crate. Since ancient times this dreadful disease has been the most feared affliction of humans so most stringent precautions were called for when handling suspect material.

At the laboratory the opening of the *debe*, the removal of the two halves of the brain, the subsequent handling and disposal or sterilisation of the tissues and potentially contaminated materials, such as goggles and overalls, had to be performed with aseptic precautions. The establishment of a positive diagnosis depends on the finding of tiny inclusion bodies called Negri bodies within certain cells of the brain when thin ribbon-like sections of brain have been mounted on miscoscope slides and then stained with an appropriate dye.

It is a rather selfish relief to find several well-formed, clearly stained Negri bodies as soon as one looks down the microscope. That's it, the job is done! Sadly, although I had seen positive slides in the pathology classes at college, I could not convince myself that there were any in that one, my first suspected case in the real world. Had we done the staining properly, how long should I keep on searching? Difficult questions, particularly under the watchful eyes of my new assistants. In Tanganyika, however, the delays involved in getting the suspect brain to the lab meant that the doctor in charge of a patient who had been bitten seldom waited for the results before submitting the patient to the ordeal of being given the Pasteur vaccine. It was the only treatment/preventive measure then available to destroy the virus before it completed its journey along the nerves from the bite mark or other point of entry to the brain where it brought on the appalling symptoms. Even the vaccination was an ordeal for the patient as it involved painful injections across the abdomen on fourteen consecutive days. Furthermore, there was always a slight risk of post-vaccination paralysis occurring in patients treated with the chemically complex Pasteur vaccine. Though the risk was admittedly slight, death from post-vaccination paralysis was particularly tragic in cases in which the laboratory tests had subsequently shown that rabies was not involved. Irrespective of these considerations, however, the veterinary officer at the other end of the line had to have a diagnosis one way or the other before deciding whether or not to institute stringent control measures such as the tracing and destruction of in-contact animals, wherever possible. Therefore, in doubtful cases further tests had to be done.

In those days the best follow-up was the intracranial inoculation of a tiny suspension of brain tissue into laboratory mice. This was no time to risk displaying further ineptitude to those assisting me so I was somewhat relieved to find that we had neither a mouse nor sufficiently tiny needles for the purpose. I settled for a couple of rabbits, the next most suscepti-ble species within the range of laboratory animals. I did so reluctantly as it was not pleasant having to submit innocent creatures to the danger of such a dreadful fate or to burden myself with the risks of keeping animals possibly incubating such a deadly virus confined in makeshift isolation premises. Fortunately for all concerned, neither of the rabbits died of either mechanically inflicted brain damage or rabies.

The laboratory dealt with a great many other specimens from our own herds and flocks, and from the field, for diagnostic procedures much less complicated and stressful than the above. Much of this routine work was handled very competently by the laboratory assistants. However, the really important work, almost the *raison d'être* of the laboratory was the production of rinderpest vaccine, just as the control of the disease in the field was the primary preoccupation of the whole Department. Its responsibility in this regard to the vast territories to the south was indeed onerous. To understand the significance of this responsibility it is necessary to consider briefly the history of the devastation that this plague created in Africa during the first half of the twentieth century.

As mentioned earlier, rinderpest is a highly fatal contagious disease of great antiquity that ravaged the cattle populations of Europe, Asia and the Indian subcontinent during the greater part of the last two millennia. The last epizootic took place in Western Europe in the 1870s but the disease has persisted even to the present time in parts of Asia, the Indian subcontinent and parts of Africa south of the Sahara. Despite this, apart from a few self-limiting outbreaks in Egypt, it did not establish itself in Africa until near the end of the nineteenth century. It is not clear whether it spread slowly southward from Egypt or first gained entrance to East Africa through the importation of Indian cattle into Somaliland in 1887 or 1889. In any event, it was present in Uganda and Masailand in 1890 (perhaps somewhat earlier) where it decimated herds of cattle and many species of indigenous antelopes. Populations of cattle that have never been exposed to the virus are highly susceptible and it is likely that more than ninety per cent of the affected cattle were wiped out as the plague swept southwards through East Africa. Lugard, in describing the mortalities in Masailand stated that "never before in the memory of man, or by the voice of tradition, have cattle died in such numbers; never before has the wild game suffered. Nearly all the buffalo and eland are gone". The Masai, who as pastoralists lived almost exclusively on the blood and milk of their cattle, were decimated. It has been suggested that perhaps half the

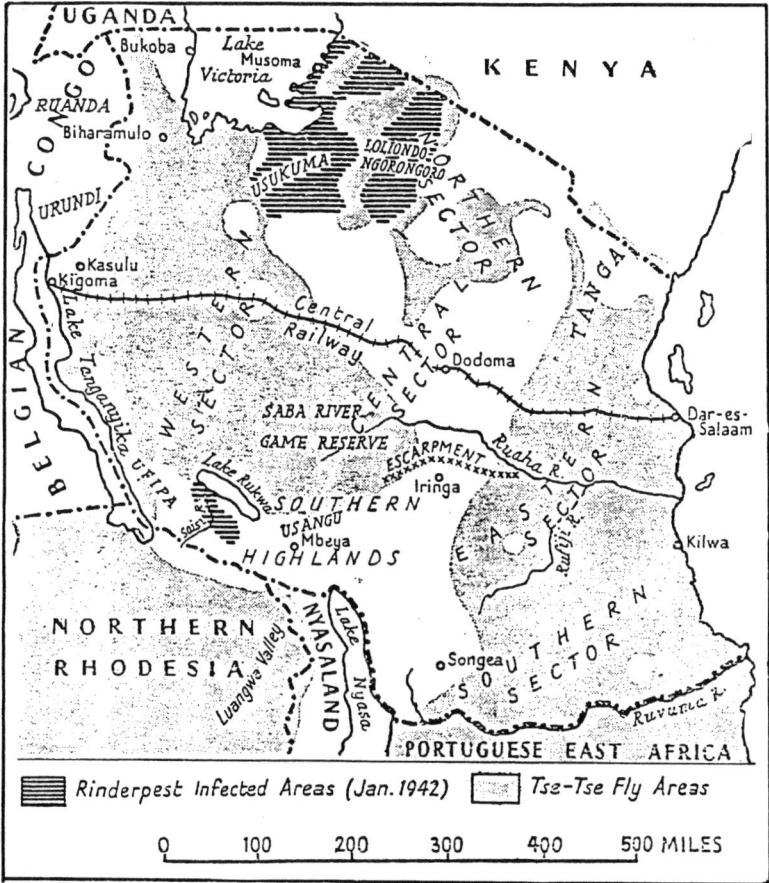

Map showing the circuitous route, heavily stocked with cattle, between tsetse infested bush to the east and to the west that constituted a potential corridor for the transmission of rinderpest down to South Africa.

Masai of Tanganyika, who lived in what was then called the German sphere of influence, starved to death because they were quite incapable of cultivating food crops as a substitute diet.

Two years later rinderpest reached southern Tanganyika in the general vicinity of the northern tip of Lake Nyasa. This was the gateway to South Africa. Early in 1896 large numbers of cattle were dying on both sides of the Zambezi River. From there it raced through Matabeleland which Rhodes had acquired for himself as part of his private colony –

now Zimbabwe. As described by Thomas Packenham, 'By March 1896 it was heading for Bulawayo, killing the transport oxen dead in their tracks and leaving a trail of stinking carcasses along every road. The authorities panicked'. The losses inflicted on the cattle-loving Ndebele people, coupled with the futile, high-handed efforts taken by Rhodes' people to control the disease was one of the major factors that triggered the Matabele rebellion which exploded almost immediately and soon spread to Mashonaland. No quarter was given on either side. Two hundred and forty-four whites – men, women and children were hacked to death. Few prisoners were taken by the whites; instead, the blacks were shot down in their hundreds as they fled.

Nothing could stop rinderpest's southern advance into the Transvaal. Desperate efforts were taken to halt its spread, including the erection of a wire fence almost a thousand miles long from the south-western corner of Bechuanaland to the Indian Ocean south of Durban. Nevertheless, the disease was carried through into Cape Colony in 1897.

Fortunately, at this point a primitive procedure for immunising cattle had been found. It consisted of injecting the bile of naturally or artificially infected animals into susceptible cattle and, despite its many limitations, the arrival of this crude vaccine marked the turning point in the fight against the disease. Concurrently, other work was in progress which resulted in the development of a more refined procedure involving the simultaneous inoculation of hyperimmune serum and virulent blood. Consequently, in less than two years more than two million cattle had been immunised by one or other of these procedures and by 1905 rinderpest had been eradicated from South Africa. Nevertheless, by then rinderpest, in that area alone, had killed more than two-and-a-half million cattle, an untold number of game animals and it had inflicted appalling hardship on the cattle owners as well as immense damage to the economy. The disease was eventually eradicated or just disappeared from all the countries south of Tanganyika through which it had swept from 1892 onwards, but for many, many years thereafter outbreaks continued to occur throughout Tanganyika and in the countries to the north.

Eventually it was agreed by international convention that Tanganyika would assume responsibility for containing the disease north of the Central Railway line running for some seven hundred miles from

Dar es Salaam to Kigoma on Lake Tanganyika. Immediately south of the line at Mpwapwa there was a corridor of relatively open country, about two hundred miles wide, heavily stocked with cattle, that led by a circuitous route down to the gap between the southern end of Lake Tanganyika and the northern tip of Lake Nyasa - the gateway to South Africa. The corridor was flanked to the east and the west by tsetse-fly-infested bush. (See Plate X.) Although cattle could not survive in tsetse bush populations of game animals, notably antelopes and buffalo which are susceptible to rinderpest, can do so with impunity. When outbreaks of rinderpest broke out in cattle in contact with susceptible game the disease was liable to be transmitted to the latter which then carried the virus into tsetse bush where it could smoulder on for prolonged periods, sometimes perhaps indefinitely. Consequently, the cattle country south of the railway line was a tinderbox for the disease.

While circumscribed outbreaks in cattle could be snuffed out by a combination of quarantine and immunisation, the only defence against the disease in game was surveillance of the game, particularly in the vast areas of tsetse bush lying to the west and the east of the more open cattle country. This was attempted by the establishment of an intelligence service headed by expatriate game rangers supported by African game scouts, who were all members of the Department of Veterinary Science and Animal Husbandry.

Sadly, recruitment came to an end during the Great Recession of the thirties and as World War Two approached staff numbers had been depleted by retrenchment and retirements. Serious outbreaks occurred south of the railway line in 1938, 1939 and 1941. They were brought under control by strenuous efforts with the help of veterinary personnel from Nyasaland, Northern and Southern Rhodesia and the Union of South Africa. For instance, during 1940 it was decided to immunise all of the cattle south of the railway line right down to the Nyalaland-Rhodesian-Tanganyika border and to intensify the intelligence service in both cattle and game areas.

To ease the logistical difficulties a field laboratory was set up at high speed for the production of the 'Mpwapwa vaccine' in an expropriated German coffee plantation, twenty miles north of the border, whose owner had been interned. During the course of the campaign groups of susceptible cattle were artificially infected with the virus and five days later slaughtered for recovery of the spleen and lymph nodes from which the vaccine was made. In total four thousand head of cattle were slaughtered, sometimes at the rate of one hundred per day, to yield a total of 13,000 litres of vaccine. The effective isolation of so many infected animals and the sterilisation of the cadavers and equipment under primitive field conditions called for the exercise of remarkable ingenuity.

During the six month campaign one million six hundred inoculations were administered to cattle widely distributed over a vast tract of country extending from Mpwapwa down to the Nyasaland/Northern Rhodesia border. This was no mean task, given the primitive infrastructure of the country at the time. As recorded by the Director of Veterinary Services:

> 'continual rain made safari and inoculation a nightmare, and the indescribably wet and filthy conditions called for heroic efforts on the part of both field and laboratory staff. In addition to these discomforts the intelligence service had to make and keep contact with the herds of game, a duty which requires courage and perseverance, more especially when dealing with sick game animals which are often really dangerous'.

As the war progressed the authorities became increasingly worried that the disease might break through once again to South Africa. Apart from the dire economic consequences for the whole of the southern half of the continent, South Africa was a vital source of tinned beef for the British and Commonwealth forces fighting in the desert and subsequently in the Far East.

The rinderpest situation deteriorated seriously during 1944. There were serious outbreaks in the Western, Lake, Northern and Tanga Provinces. In May of that year there was an outbreak, the first ever, on Zanzibar Island though it was quickly eradicated by mass immunisation. The situation was much more worrying on the mainland because the disease smouldered on in game in certain areas where it had been brought under control by quarantine and immunisation. The immune status of the cattle population south of the Central Railway line which had been immunised in 1940 was now negligible, because of the limited longevity of the immunity induced by the Mpwapwa vaccine as well as the recruitment of successive generations of completely susceptible calves into the herds. Similarly, the immune status of game animals that had earlier been exposed to the virus would have been diluted by their immunologically naive progeny.

Consequently, when I took over the laboratory my over-riding concern was my responsibility for the safekeeping of the stock of live virus kept in a fridge for the inoculation of susceptible cattle during the course of vaccine production. As far as we were aware, Mpwapwa was the most southerly location of the virus in Africa. There we were, with highly susceptible cattle in our immediate vicinity and literally hundreds of thousands south of the railway line only twelve miles from Mpwapwa. This was my constant preoccupation because cattle were artificially infected with the virus practically every week during the course of vaccine production.

The first step in the process of vaccine production was the transfer of a group of up to twenty rinderpest-susceptible cattle into a concrete-floored shed in the rinderpest *boma* where they were allowed to settle down. During this period they were temperatured daily and then injected with virulent blood that had been collected from the previously infected group. Almost invariably, the body temperature rose above normal on the third day after infection and was well up by the fifth. At this point the animal was slaughtered and a thorough post-mortem examination conducted to confirm that the fever was actually due to rinderpest. This was done by finding the diagnostic lesions at various points in the alimentary tract. In those days, long before the development of the ultra microscope, the virus was invisible even under the highest power of the light microscope, so the characteristic temperature reaction in conjunction with the post-mortem lesions was taken on faith - and reliably so - as evidence that the virus had multiplied exceedingly during the five days.

Superficial lymph nodes and the spleen were removed aseptically and transferred to the laboratory where they were passed through an ordinary mincing machine. The pulp was diluted one in four with glycerine containing 0.1 per cent formalin. Next day, the viscid brew was filled into sterile beer bottles that were then sealed with ordinary crown caps. A week later, the vaccine was considered 'mature' and safe for dispatch to the field.

It was always good to walk through the vaccine laboratory on a Saturday morning. The cheery activity of the attendants passing a continuous line of beer bottles, hand over hand, to the crown cap machine operator who swung the lever up and down to the accompaniment of the clatter of bottles and light-hearted banter from all present was a very satisfying end to yet another busy week. But our senior Veterinary Guard, Ibrahim, a dignified utterly reliable Somali gentleman, would be still busily engaged with his gang in the rinderpest *boma* disinfecting the premises and disposing of the carcasses, the final task in the whole undertaking. For obvious reasons, stringent measures had to be taken to ensure that live virus was not allowed to escape from the *boma*. The first barrier was the confined shed in which the animals incubating the disease were housed. The second was the high perimeter brick wall surrounding the whole compound. The precautions required to prevent infection being carried out by personnel leaving the enclosure were, of course, strictly enforced. The copious excreta and ingesta of the infected animals, as well as the washings of the concrete floors, presented a particular problem. The former, stacked in heaps, and the latter, stored in tanks, were held within the *boma* for a prescribed period to ensure that they were no longer infective.

The most laborious task was the disposal of the carcasses. They had to be dismembered and every bit boiled thoroughly in great cauldrons over wood fires in a corner of the *boma* to destroy the virus. The spectacle of the labourers applying their knives and machetes to the carcasses, against a background of billowing steam from the cauldrons and smoke from the wood fires was like a scene from Dante's Inferno. One regretted that the remains of each of these animals, which had been obliged to make the supreme sacrifice in order to save the lives of some 250 of their unknown kin, might not have been disposed of with greater delicacy! However, we lived in a practical world and the carcasses had to be cleared as quickly as possible to make way for the next batch of susceptibles.

It was also a fact of life that our labourers and the populace in general lived with an ever-present shortage of animal protein. Generous helpings of meat, even well-boiled rinderpest meat, were a great treat so there was no difficulty in arranging for long lines of our labourers and others in the know to queue up in good time on 'rinderpest meat days' for its orderly distribution. The distribution of the meat represented the end of the process and cleared the decks for the admission of another batch of susceptible cattle to the rinderpest *boma* when necessary.

Although the Mpwapwa vaccine was rather crude, more expensive and much bulkier than the Kabete Attenuated Goat Virus Vaccine (KAG), which was then available from Kenya and coming into use on a large scale, the Tanganyika Department set great store by the former. While the immunological mechanism of the Mpwapwa vaccine was not clearly understood it was safer and more reliable than KAG for cattle under one year so it was reserved for such animals. Though dearer than KAG it was still cost-effective since an average-sized donor bullock yielded approximately 250 doses of vaccine. It was also an advantage, particularly in wartime, that no imported ingredients other than glycerine and a modicum of formaldehyde were required for its manufacture.

While vaccine production, supervision of routine diagnostic work and the Acting C.V.R.O's experiments and administration occupied most of my time, the farm work outside the laboratory buildings, apart from the purely veterinary activities, was in the capable hands of the Acting Livestock Officer and one of the Apprentice Stock Inspectors. This consisted mainly of the management of the two experimental dairy farms, including the recording of milk yields and other data; the management of the other herds and flocks; weekly dipping of all the cattle; cultivation of fodder crops, hay making, bush clearing and the improvement and extension of grassland. The latter involved an endless battle against regenerating bush on the established pastures and the planting of newly cleared areas with star grass. A large team of labourers was employed continuously for the monotonous work of bush clearing by hand.

It was always refreshing to escape from the routine of the lab when a little clinical work had to be done. The limitations of the drugs available in those days generally, and in wartime Tanganyika in particular, were at times frustrating. Sulphanilamide was the only antibiotic available for the treatment of a limited range of bacterial infections. Anaesthesia was primitive compared with the present state of the art and too often had to be substituted by restraint. This rendered surgical intervention unpleasant and, at times, hazardous. For example, we had a particularly aggressive warthog well equipped with vicious tusks in a concrete floored pen in the zoo. It did not have enough exercise to wear down the hooves of its hind legs. They grew rapidly and a month or two after I had taken over they were curving upwards in a semi-circle and needed attention. The zoo keeper kept reminding me of the fact but this irritated me because, frankly, I was scared. How wonderful to have had one of today's anaesthetic dart guns! Eventually, it dawned on me to ask the attendant how "Bwana Wildie" (the Ag.C.V.R.O.) had done the job last time. The procedure was both simple and effective. We starved the warthog for a day or two and at the appointed time when all was ready the brave keeper entered the cage with a large dish of sloppy grub in one hand and a hurdle in the other. Once the warthog began to eat the attendant used the hurdle to ease its backside over to the bars where I was ready with a large funnel with a length of rubber tubing attached containing a warm solution of the sedative chloral hydrate. From my side of the bars I gently inserted the well-oiled end of the tube through the anus of the warthog into the rectum. We all held our breath as another attendant slowly raised the funnel higher and higher as the prescribed dose passed in at an even pace. In due course, the erstwhile wicked warthog settled down like a somnolent old gentleman after a hearty lunch at the club, whereupon I was in like a flash with a pair of shears to perform the chiropody in record time.

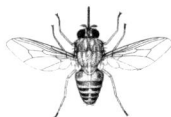

CHAPTER TEN

A Bachelor's Ménage

With the departure of Mac's entourage the author's servants develop a proprietary interest in the household. Last boxes are unpacked, photos and other treasures soften the decor. Entertaining is encouraged to compete with established households. RAF guests on leave from the humid heat of the coast fill the house with ribald laughter.

After Mac left for Singida the rest house was ours alone so we completed the unpacking and put our own stamp on the humble surroundings. *Mpishi* had gone to Dar es Salaam to fetch his wife so there was only Selemani to share my pleasure in displaying the few civilising elements that my mother and dear sisters had pressed on me, such as cushion covers, colourful antimacassars, table-cloths, some silver and family photographs. They softened not only the sitting room but also my own feelings because the faces in the photos, with the exception of my brother's, were still about three months away by air mail. All I knew about my brother was that he was "somewhere at sea" on the HMS *Fencer*, c/o The GPO, London! When *Mpishi* returned with his wife he brought with him what proved to be the room's crowning glory, a sparkling new multi-coloured sisal carpet. With this in place *Mpishi* insisted that it was quite improper for a *Bwana mganga wa wanyama* (a veterinary surgeon) to live without curtains, even though there was mosquito netting on the windows. But curtain material was unobtainable. Selemani did not consider this a problem and he managed to find a roll of jute sacking and some purple Drummers Dye in the village. The jute, which was probably imported from India, was in plentiful supply. A picture comes back to me of Selemani enveloped in a cloud of steam as he applied a pole to lengths of sacking in a boiling cauldron with his white hat still hanging on precariously to the back of his perspiring head. He was delighted with the results; *Mpishi*, unsmiling as usual, expressed his approval with a solemn nod when the first curtain was hung.

Before long the 'boys' began to teach me manners. With no little shop nearer than the village, provisions were bought in bulk and it was customary when starting with a new staff to lock the store cupboard and hand out rations every few days. But life was so busy that breakfasts, not to mention rations, were the last thing I thought of as I shot past Selemani at seven o'clock every morning on my way to the lab. On one occasion when I returned for breakfast more than ready for a lovely plate of porridge and cream it was solemnly served by Selemani who then hovered expectantly until I exclaimed, 'What - no salt!' He was ready for it, 'Sorry Bwana, you forget to leave the salt for *Mpishi*'. A few days later the usual freshly baked loaf was missing - '*Mpishi* had no flour, Bwana'! At dinner otherwise excellent banana fritters or fruit salads were likely to be sugarless. Before long the carefully co-ordinated strategy wore me down. The store cupboard was thrown open, breakfasts were once again accompanied by smiles and jokes and thereafter all that was required to discourage excessive filching was an occasional remark from me that we seemed to be getting through a particular grocery rather quickly.

The cook was relieved that his wife had settled down and some days after her arrival he suggested that I should send to *Ulaya* (England) for mine. I refrained from explaining that I was a bachelor; instead I brushed it off by saying that it was impossible during wartime. After dinner that night Selemani was in a talkative mood. He bent over the family photographs and asked if my brother was an *askari* (soldier) and proceeded to extract a lot of the family history. Lastly he picked up the photo of my youngest sister and asked if she was my *bibi* (wife). I explained that I was a bachelor, whereupon he withdrew smartly and hurried down to the kitchen where I overheard him delivering the *habari* (news) to *Mpishi* and his *bibi*. When he returned with the coffee he diffidently muttered that *Mpishi* and he missed their friends and the food at Dar es Salaam; that they disliked Mpwapwa because it was too cold; there was no fish and rice was expensive. He went on to acknowledge that I was a good Bwana, that the cold of Mpwapwa was good for me and there was little fever. Nevertheless, they prayed every day that I would not get sick because such matters were a *shauri la Mungu* (affair of God). They were going to stay and look after me. I was rather touched; clearly the food rationing had been forgiven though at the back of my mind I just wondered if they were working up to negotiate a rise in pay or to sell me a *bibi*. It was a great comfort to have such a reliable pair and before long they got their rise, but the need for bride price never arose.

By and large, the Tanganyikans, even in those days of colonial rule, were a most likeable, admirable people - gentle, kind and courteous. These characteristics were undoubtedly an integral part of their nature, not just a sycophantic response to the relative wealth and authority of the whites. The benign interracial relationship, so much at variance with the situation in many other dependant territories, was facilitated by the political status of the country. Following the defeat of German East Africa by the British Forces in 1918 the actual territory became Tanganyika Territory in 1922 and its administration was formally handed over in trust to Great Britain by the League of Nations as a mandated territory. While the British Government presumably saw advantages to itself in accepting this arrangement the indigenous people also benefited greatly by escaping from the harsh rule of the previous administration. After the handover they were treated much more benevolently. For example, while the limited areas that had been occupied by German settlers passed into the hands of a relatively small number of nationalities such as British, Greeks and Indians there was no further expropriation of land. The country was no longer a colony so there were no opportunities for further settlement. Consequently, the vast majority of the expatriates were civil servants, birds of passage, with no vested interest in the country other than their jobs, and a pension for those who chose to stay on to the age of fifty-five.

Looking on as a bachelor, I could see that those who were married and had committed themselves to the country paid a high price for the security, such as it was, of their jobs and the admitted satisfaction that they obtained from their work. Their wives were obliged to live in considerable discomfort, particularly up-country, with limited opportunity to choose congenial female company. The benefits they derived from abundant domestic help left more time on their hands and aggravated their loneliness. Children were sent, at about the age of six, for schooling in Kenya or Europe and in the latter case wives were torn between being separated from their children or from their husbands. Couples who committed themselves in those days to the long haul with a pension at fifty-five did so in the knowledge that on retirement they would face the stress of settling down in Europe or elsewhere in changed surroundings just at the time when their offspring were scattering. I soon reckoned it was no place for family life. Selemani's and *Mpishi*'s urging me to send home for a *bibi* would have carried little weight with me even if it had been possible for me to do so.

For the moment, but only for the moment, the company of other bachelors, of which there was no shortage, compensated reasonably well. Variety was provided by visitors from an RAF base at Dar es Salaam who were offered hospitality at Mpwapwa. The pleasure they displayed at escaping from the humid heat of the coast and experiencing, often for the first time, what most of us considered to be the real Africa, was stimulating for us as was their enjoyment of the freedom and culinary delights of even a bachelor's household after months in barracks. For the host it was delightful to get news and fresh jokes from beyond our mountain fastness and to have the monastic silence of a bachelor abode replaced by ribald laughter.

On the eve of the expected arrival of my first pair of RAF visitors *Mpishi*, Selemani and I had to deal with a minor crisis. At that early stage I had not managed to acquire a fridge so it was a tricky business providing a daily supply of meat. The lab killed a bullock once a week for the benefit of the expatriate and senior African staff, which was fine for households with fridges. Whether one had a fridge or not, most households kept a few chickens, one of which could be made oven-ready at the drop of a hat. Indeed, there was a story in circulation to the effect that when visitors from bush blew in unexpectedly to a particular house just before dinner a message was shouted down the garden by the house boy to the cook, '*Wageni wamefika, chinga kuku na tia maji indani ya soupu*' ('strangers have arrived, kill a chicken and put water into the soup'). Note how every word in Swahili ends in a vowel, giving the language a lovely cadence.

In our own crisis *Mpishi* announced that the meat had gone off and we had eaten our last chicken. I told him not to worry, that I would go out that afternoon and shoot a couple of guineafowl. At that precise moment

Selemani was on his knees with his head in a cupboard searching for something. I heard a muffled '*labda*'. He knew my Swahili was still very shaky but he did not realise that I knew that '*labda*', especially in the way he said it, meant 'yeah, perhaps'. Admittedly, he was being perspicacious because the Apprentice Stock Inspector, Phillip Princello, who was my constant companion on our frequent shooting expeditions, and I had come back empty-handed from a series of recent outings. This was now a point of honour so I took one of the horses and went a considerable distance to join Phillip at a spot where he had set up camp in connection with a particular job. Coming from an Africander family that had settled in Northern Tanganyika he was an experienced hunter and had located an area where guineafowl were fairly thick on the ground. We had a great afternoon and I arrived home well after dark with enough guineafowl for myself and my neighbours (see illust.). I handed a brace to Selemani and asked him as best I could in Swahili: 'What is *labda*?' With a broad grin he raised two fingers and answered, '*Kanga mbili Bwana*' (two guineafowl) and then, with a characteristic contortion, bent himself double with laughter as he staggered around the room slapping his thigh!

Our RAF visitors on this occasion proved to be great company and it was good to see how much they enjoyed their first expedition up-country after six months in the relatively suburban atmosphere of Dar es Salaam. When we took them on their first climb up Kiborani Mountain to enjoy the nostalgia of sitting in front of a blazing fire in the rest house that had been built near the top for bracing weekend breaks they brushed aside my offer of sun helmets. Apparently, RAF fitters spent most of the day scrambling over their aircraft in the full glare of Dar sunshine clad only in shorts and sunglasses. Though some of them may have regretted their excessive exposure in later years their relaxed attitude certainly put into another perspective the need for wearing red felt spine pads and sun helmets lined with silver paper, as advocated so solemnly by the Colonial Office.

Although desserts were not *Mpishi*'s strong suit the visitors enthused about the banana fritters, fruit salads and crème brulée with real cream but they did not stay long enough to realise that that was the extent of his repertoire! After their departure *Mpishi* was worn out and effortless fruit salad or a slice of pawpaw was served night after night. Eventually, I groaned, 'Ah no! Not another fruit salad'. Next night, Selemani shambled into the dining room with one arm awkwardly behind his back and announced '*Siku kuu, leo*' which meant 'holiday today' or 'special day'. When I asked what on earth he was talking about, he swung his arm around with a contortion of the shoulders involving a laboured twist of the wrist to reveal a plate, still balancing upright in the palm of his hand, and giggled 'Fruitie saladie, Bwana'. Even a bachelor's house was never dull with a fellow like him around!

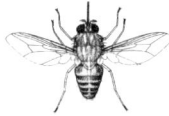

CHAPTER ELEVEN

Stress and Strain

An outbreak of the deadly disease African swine fever in hundreds of pigs at a bizarre bacon factory miles from Mpwapwa adds to the pressure. Tensions in Head Office and the Lab relating to rinderpest cause a short, sharp shindy between the Director and the author.

The Director of Veterinary Services, Bertie Lowe, was a remarkable man. He had been with the Department since its very beginning, having been released from the Royal Army Veterinary Corps, at the request of the Colonial office, immediately after the end of the First World War. He was one of the first two veterinary officers to report for duty at Dar es Salaam on 13 December 1918. Thereupon, he was sent to Dodoma, right in the centre of the country, to consult with the District Political Officers as to how best his services could be used. Failure of the rains had brought famine, influenza was rampant and people were dying. In short, his civilian career began in bush with few, if any, resources at his disposal, rather than behind a desk at Dar es Salaam. During the next twenty years his dynamic personality enabled him to acquire an intimate knowledge of the whole country at the coal-face and a profound understanding of its problems and its people, with whom he had lived for months on end while on foot safari. By the time he became Director of Veterinary Services in 1938 he was uniquely well qualified for the post by virtue of his hands-on experience and his innate leadership qualities. His management of the catastrophic rinderpest situation in southern Tanganyika from 1938 to 1941, following its escape across the Central Railway line, earned him the respect and confidence of the various countries to the south of Tanganyika.

Though short in stature, he was a big man in every sense of the word, well-known internationally, affectionately respected by his staff, unmistakably the boss, rather fierce when roused but charming and immensely kind when the necessity arose, and tolerant of the naivety of youngsters. I must admit, I was rather pleased that he was Irish and, as such, was a graduate of the Dublin Veterinary College. By long-established tradition students sat in alphabetical order in lecture theatres in their early years so I may even have sat in the same row, if not the actual seat, that he had occupied some thirty years earlier. And there we were, both in Mpwapwa!

But no favours were shown! Understandably, he was obviously worried that I might not be able to cope, so after Mac left he called to the lab most mornings before breakfast. It became my job to escort him on tours of different facilities, chosen by him at random. It was like a military inspection and as we entered each facility the staff stood up respectfully with a '*Jambo asabui Bwana Mkubwa*' (Good morning big Bwana). The '*Mkubwa*' was reserved for him. I escorted him with trepidation, never knowing what terrible evidence of neglect or incompetence might lie around the next corner. Indeed, in the early days the click, click of his walking stick approaching along the veranda was enough to interrupt abruptly any discussion taking place in my office. But I soon began to value these regular inspections. They were a disciplined way of keeping in touch with what was going on and, of course, I learnt much from the Director during our joint perambulations. As time went on the visitations became progressively less frequent and eventually petered out when pressures from outside began to bear down on both of us.

Rinderpest, in a mild form that was difficult to diagnose, was smouldering in Tabora District almost on the Central Railway line. A big immunisation campaign was in progress in the Central Province and a particularly virulent strain of the virus was killing cattle and game near Tanga. It was a worrying time for the Director with a depleted staff in the field and only a youngster in the lab. Life was not easy for the latter either. One morning the Director phoned to tell me that they needed all the vaccine they could get their hands on and asked how much I could make during the next month. Thinking aloud, I assured him that we had plenty of susceptibles at Matamondo but the most we could safely accommodate in the rinderpest hospital was twenty per week. I was immediately told to double them up. No discussion!

One Sunday morning thereafter, with the rinderpest hospital full to the gunnels, a battered aluminium-bodied car drove up to my house. A dumpy, elderly man climbed out and walked up to the veranda, shoulders stooped, head thrown forward, arms spread wide with fingers unclenched hanging loosely as if to get the maximum cooling effect from any breeze going - obviously a man who had spent most of his life outdoors in the African sun. This was Tom Bain but he was so much a part of the country that he was referred to by most people as Bwana Bain. He lived with his wife and sister-in-law on the side of a mountain away out in bush near the little village of Mlali, fifty miles away. He came to German East Africa from Southern Rhodesia during the First World War and eventually returned to Tanganyika in 1919 where he made a living from mica mining although he was one of those people who could turn his hand to anything. During the Second World War he established a pig farm and bacon factory at Mlali for the production of bacon and sausages which had previously been imported from Kenya and further afield. Mlali was an ideal location for the purpose as it had an unfailing supply of spring water from the side of a mountain for the factory and ample unused land on which to grow feed for the pigs under irrigation. Though it was isolated this posed no real problem for pioneers like the Bains. Even during the rains they seldom failed to make the journey of more than sixty miles into the railway station at Gulwe, laden with baskets of bacon and vegetables neatly labelled for their customers all along the line. There were practically no other pigs elsewhere in Central Province and only seven thousand in the whole country. Consequently, the arrival of the treasured commodity added greatly to the pleasure of Europeans and others living near the wayside stops. It was a custom to wander down to the station, as soon as the toot of the approaching train was heard, to meet friends in transit and to hear news of the outside world.

Bwana Bain had the carcasses of three fine baconers in the back of the car. Twelve others, out of a total of several hundred, had died suddenly during the course of the previous twenty-four hours. He was a very worried man, so we lost no time in getting them up to the lab. The only history he could give was that some were found dead, while others merely showed listlessness, inappetance and arching of the back, which was suggestive of pain, before dying within twenty-four hours. Having eliminated the possibility of anthrax we opened the carcasses and found intensely red patches and ulcers in the mouth and intense haemmorrhagic inflammation of the stomach and intestines. It was obviously essential to see the herd. The Director was away so I called on Neil Reid, the Senior Veterinary Officer at Headquarters, to seek permission. A kindly, fatherly man, he was always happy to pass on the fruits of his long experience in the field to the younger generation. He urged me to go immediately as he recognised that it might just be African swine fever, an even more serious variant of the disease that in those days was a major hazard to pig farming elsewhere in the world. The African variant occurred in a hyper-acute form and had a mortality rate of almost one hundred per cent.

The first part of the thirty-five mile journey to Bwana Bain's was a refreshing escape from the narrow confines of Mpwapwa. The rains had just started and the previously dry thorn bush was already a delicate green. We made good time for the first twelve miles to Matamonda where we kept our reserve herd of rinderpest-susceptible cattle. From that point on we began to climb slowly uphill across the mountains. At several points where the road had been washed away Bwana Bain's boy and I had to hack out and lay a carpet of bush poles and push the vehicle, metaphor-ically keeping our fingers crossed that it would do the trick. This stretch was uninhabited. The damp mountain air was getting chilly and the prospect of being stuck there overnight until some foot travellers passed by was uninviting. The sun was low on the horizon when we broke out of the trees on our descent at the other side of the mountain and saw before us a vast, empty plain stretching to the north, east and west as far as the eye could see. This was the real Africa after the confinement of Mpwapwa. From there we sped eastwards, following our rapidly length-ening shadow, along the plain to the village of Mlali where groups of children and adults cheered us on our way to the Bains' shamba up the side of a nearby hill. The sun had just dipped below the horizon as we were greeted by Bwana Bain's ladies who had watched our approach from the veranda of their spartan, tin-roofed house. Spartan though it was the house was aglow with electric light amid the surrounding darkness. Bwana Bain, being the man he was, had long since harnessed the water cascading down the hill behind the house to a generator for the factory and his own comfort. All of this, and hundreds of pigs, in the middle of a wilderness some thirty miles away from the nearest Europeans who were located at a mission station near the tiny village of Kongwa. That village, I later witnessed, was to become famous in less than two years as the bustling headquarters of the ill-fated Groundnut Scheme. For the moment the talk over a welcome pot of tea was all about pigs. Another five baconers had died during the day but as it was now dark nothing could be done until morning.

The growing pigs were kept outdoors in paddocks holding different age groups. The baconers were in a number of enclosures on flatter ground further away from the house and so far the deaths had been confined to one of these groups. This leaned one towards African swine fever as it was generally believed that wild pigs and warthogs served as carriers of the virus which was easily transmitted to domestic pigs by indirect contact when the opportunity arose. This seemed the only way it could have been introduced to Bwana Bain's herd as there were no other domestic pigs within a hundred miles. There had been no deaths overnight and apart from a few individuals showing listlessness and floppy ears there was nothing very spectacular to be seen, so it was decided to do autopsies on those that had died the previous day before the carcasses deteriorated. After breakfast we would temperature as many as possible because in African swine fever the first symptom, sometimes the only significant one, is a high fever.

The autopsies showed the same intense haemorrhagic inflammation of the stomach and intestines as we had seen at the lab. After breakfast we began temperaturing. It was not an easy job as there were about fifty well-grown pigs with plenty of space in the affected paddock. We erected a makeshift pen in one corner. A superfluity of labourers herded as many pigs as possible towards the pen but it was a messy business with a mass of pigs screeching, as only indignant pigs can. The high-pitched cacophony was punctuated by the shouting of unduly excited attendants in hot pursuit of a succession of individuals that broke ranks and belted down the paddock to join earlier escapees. Two or three of the more trustworthy attendants stood outside our little pen to grab the nearest pig as required and to manhandle it struggling into the presence of Bwana Bain, with notepad poised, and me with thermometer in hand. My job was to ease the thermometer into the rectum of each resentful pig. The whole thing was a vigorous, dusty and sweaty undertaking.

The rectal temperatures of the first few were within the normal range (*circa* 102' F) but then readings of up to 106' F began to crop up all too frequently. I had never seen swine fever before, but this was very worrying. Bwana Bain was even more worried - he too was aware of the high mortality associated with African swine fever, as well as the fact that there was absolutely no effective treatment or vaccine available anywhere for the disease.

During our gloomy deliberations over a late lunch Bwana Bain, practical man that he was, came up with a suggestion that impressed me greatly. He was prepared to settle for swine fever, or for some other unknown highly infectious disease, but even if all the in-contact baconers died he was determined to salvage as many as possible of the other baconers and younger stock. He proposed to divide all the different categories of pigs into groups of about twenty-five each and to set up new, well-separated paddocks some distance out in bush - there was no shortage of empty land as far as the eye could see - and transfer each group to a separate enclosure. In this way he hoped that groups in which none of the individuals had been incubating the infection at the time of transfer would be saved. I have to admit that such a scheme would never have occurred to me because I was still conditioned by the stereotyped methods of control practised at home. Had swine fever broken out in Ireland, as it did some years later, there would have been banner headlines in the national newspapers, excitement in the Department of Agriculture with veterinary inspectors falling over themselves, quarantine and slaughter of the affected herd or herds, disinfection of premises and prohibition of movement of pigs over extensive areas.

I had slight reservations about the post-mortem lesions and was reluctant to take heroic measures immediately. Putting the whole herd out to bush even in widely dispersed enclosures incurred the risk of exposing, at least, some groups to wild pigs or warthogs possibly carrying the virus. Word came that another baconer had died in the group investigated that morning. A post-mortem examination on this fine fresh carcass showed the same lesions - intense haemorrhagic inflammation of the gastro-intestinal tract – so we decided to inject some blood into three weaners placed in strict isolation indoors. If it was acute African swine fever, temperatures should be up in three or four days. We decided to temperature the baconers again and, to our intense surprise, practically all were within the normal range with only a few up to 104' F. I suddenly realised what a fool I had been and, indeed, Bwana Bain might have known better. It was now the cool of the evening and it dawned on me that before lunch we had merely been driving the unfortunate pigs to higher and higher temperatures as our exertions progressed in the midday sun! 'Mad dogs and Englishmen!'

As we wandered round the paddock in the fading light, uncertain as to whether we should disperse the healthy pigs out in bush at the risk of exposing them to infected warthogs, we happened to see broken soil at the base of a cactus-like tree where pigs had been rooting. The same was seen at the rest of these trees within the paddock. I was soon informed that the roots and the green branches when cut exuded a milky white sap which was 'moto sana' (very hot) and was used by witch doctors as medicine. This further eroded our provisional diagnosis of swine fever. Since I had to return to Mpwapwa early next morning we decided that Bwana Bain should set up a completely new paddock on ground free of the cactus-like trees and well away from the existing paddocks. All the pigs from the affected paddock would be transferred there, as soon as possible. In the meantime, Bwana Bain would keep his eyes on the three weaners that had been injected and use his discretion as to whether he should or should not disperse all of his stock in small groups.

Early next morning I set off with a driver for Mpwapwa while Bwana Bain was already mustering labourers and gear to fence off a paddock out in bush for the pigs from the affected paddock. At Matomonda, where the lab's rinderpest-susceptible cattle were kept, we were waved down by a young African standing at the roadside on one leg in characteristic Masai posture balancing himself on his spear with the other foot pressed against the calf of the other leg. Word must have got about somehow that I was at Bwana Bain's and he had probably been waiting there since dawn. As soon as we stopped the head herdsman came running towards us from the mud huts at the side of the cattle boma. He was worried and explained that two of the cattle were sick and he thought they had rinderpest. I wished he had not even mentioned that name at a time like this! He had them penned off in the boma and they were certainly very ill and running a high temperature but the subcutaneous lymph nodes in front of the shoulders on both sides were enlarged. It seemed like East Coast fever –

I could not say 'looked like' because I had never actually seen the disease! I had only read about it. It is a fascinating disease, caused by a protozoan parasite which is transmitted by a particular species of tick. The first priority was to aspirate some lymph from one of the swollen nodes, smear it on a slide, get it back to Mpwapwa and find out what else had gone wrong during the past two days.

Back at Mpwapwa the first stop was at the laboratory where the slides were stained and put under the microscope without delay. What a joy it was to see the parasites teeming in the lymph cells in a colourful form known as Kock's bodies, called after Dr. Kock, the father of veterinary science in South Africa who first described the parasite in 1898. It did not help to have East Coast fever in our reserve of rinderpest-susceptible cattle at Mtamonda but, at least, I was relieved that it was not rinderpest itself. In due course, it was also comforting to hear from Bwana Bain that the three young pigs we had injected with suspect blood had shown no reaction whatsoever. Better still, no deaths had occurred in the baconers after they had been moved to a new cactus-free paddock. We concluded that African swine fever had not been involved.

At that point the Director returned from safari and word got around that things were rather tense in Headquarters. Almost immediately the pressures under which both he and I had been working exploded. One crisp, sunny morning I had been working up in the rinderpest *boma* with Ibrahim and his team since dawn making vaccine when a messenger arrived, out of breath and obviously distraught. He told me that Bwana Mkubwa wanted to see me in my office *mara moja*, (immediately). As soon as I arrived, the Director's florid face and reluctant greeting told me that he had already done a tour and there was trouble. He stumped off, tight-lipped, to the bacteriology laboratory with me on his heels.

The laboratory was a narrow room with just enough space for a bench and two or three stools. In this confined space he pointed to a piece of plaster that had fallen to the floor and demanded an explanation. I explained that we were so busy with the rinderpest vaccine that I had been up the previous night inoculating agar plates and on leaning back at the end of the job my stool had slipped and bashed the wall. I added that I had been in the rinderpest *boma* long before the workshops opened but undertook to attend to the matter as soon as possible. 'I see', said the

Director. We then returned to the veranda to continue our tour of inspection.

Here I should explain that one of his *bêtes noires* were *mchwa*. These are the ubiquitous white ants that have a voracious appetite for timber and an equally powerful aversion to light. Consequently, when a column emerges from the ground and climbs up the wall of a building en route to the roof timber they build a tunnel around themselves on the surface of the wall composed of tiny particles of soil cemented together by saliva. Once in the roof space the woodwork becomes encrusted with thick layers of their earthworks as they devour the timber. They work at such speed that their tunnels may extend up the wall at the rate of several feet per day. The *mchwa* are so destructive that a gentle young man, called Ugambo, doubled as laboratory animal house attendant and *mchwa fundi* (white ant expert). His duty was to go around all the buildings every day knocking *mchwa* galleries off the walls and, where practicable, pouring an insecticide down any crevices on the ground from which they were emerging.

During our silent walk along the veranda the Director stopped at a particular point and, to my horror, pointed at an earthen gallery of white ants already several feet up the wall and, tight-lipped, exclaimed, '*Mchwa, mchwa,* call that villain Ugambo'. On the arrival of a very frightened Ugambo the Director jabbed the point of his elegant walking stick into the ants' gallery and roared at Ugambo, '*Mchwa mchwa; mchwa, mchwa; namna* f---ing *gani*', with great emphasis on the 'f' word! The '*namna gani*' bit in this context means roughly 'what the hell' but an English expletive between *namna* and *gani* always has a powerful effect on the accused. Ugambo was stunned. Reacting to his obsession with *mchwa* the Director suddenly raised his stick to bash the gallery off the wall. In this context, it should be explained that it was illegal in Tanganyika for anybody to strike an African and it would, of course, have been unheard of for even a junior official, far less, a Director to do so. However, in the circumstances Ugambo was taking no chances. He happened to have arrived with a four-gallon tin *debi* in his hand and he instinctively raised it to ward of what he thought was a blow. The invitation was too great for the Director who was unable to resist the temptation. He struck the *debi* with a resounding blow and, no doubt, the excitement generated by the first metallic clang drew the two contestants immediately into a duel in which the din increased a few decibels with each successive thrust and parry. After the shock of the first bang the contest became hugely entertaining for the small group of onlookers until the ebony shaft of the walking stick suddenly separated from its ivory handle. Thereupon, Ugambo dropped the battered *debi* and immediately took to his heels as fast as his legs could take him. As the onlookers watched him disappear into bush the Director inspected his beautifully carved ivory handle and, turning to me with a quizzical smile said, quite unabashed, 'Pity Lee, that was my favourite stick!' But the mood soon changed; it was back to business.

He stalked off briskly, still holding the prized ivory in his hand, to a big shed at the back of the laboratory that was traditionally crammed with sacks of cattle feed, piles of dried ox hides waiting to be shipped, and old bits of equipment that might come in useful sometime. He pointed his stick into a crack between two rows of sacks and asked, "What's this?" I knew without looking that it was a rat trap so I explained that I had seen rat droppings recently and had set traps around the place. 'To hell with that, take a good look, Sir', he replied. I craned my neck and to my horror saw the hairs of an extremely compressed tortoiseshell cat bristling through the bars of the cage. I was annoyed. It was unfair, I had been up in the rinderpest *boma* making vaccine for him since dawn and I thought, 'this is it, he can have his flaming job, I'm off'. I looked him straight in the eyes. 'What is it?' I enunciated, then paused and spelt out slowly: 'It – is – a – cat – in –a – rat – trap'. Glancing down again I exclaimed, almost to myself, 'Oh hell, it's yours!' It must have flashed through my mind that I should seek to have other charges taken into account, so I added, 'Now Sir, I want to show you something'. This time I led the way to a shed that housed the electric generator and roared for somebody to bring the key. I threw the door open and pointed to the roof timbers completely encased in the red laterite earthworks of white ants. I said, 'Look, Sir, *mchwa*; they have been there since I took over. If I knock them down, the roof'll fall in; if I don't, the ants themselves will bring it down. What am I to do?' The Director drew his chin in with a deep intake of breath, looked down at his feet for a moment, finally inspected his watch and said 'Lee, I think it is time we both went for breakfast'.

After breakfast there was a note in the Director's handwriting lying on my desk. This was it, I was sure I was finished. I still have his note to this day! All it said was, 'Dear Lee, the cook tells me there is a nice ox tongue for dinner tonight. I should be delighted if you would care to join me.'

During the evening not a word was said about the morning's proceedings. Neither was there a sign of the tortoiseshell cat, which I imagine had been tactfully secured in more commodious confinement. From that point onwards, the Director was a great friend to me for the remainder of his service and during his all too brief retirement in Ireland. As I came to learn more and more about his achievements I began to regret the impertinence I had displayed as a callow youth, to a man of such seniority.

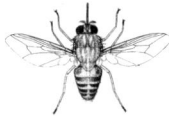

CHAPTER TWELVE

Peace in Europe, At War with Lions

News of the end of the war in Europe heard on short wave radio. Colourful local celebrations follow. A conference of Provincial Veterinary Officers considers post-war development. A famous scientist arrives to consider conducting trials with the new insecticide DDT at Mpwapwa. Attempts to kill a rampaging lion create excitement.

E ven on small stations like Mpwapwa there was a refreshing coming and going of personnel to break the monotony. For example, during the war, long leave was still granted for health reasons about every two years though it had to be taken almost invariably in South Africa because of the acute shortage of passages to and from Great Britain. Since my arrival, Van Rensburg, a new Pasture Research Officer from South Africa had arrived. Jim Buckley, known as CJ, a debonair Livestock Officer in his mid-forties returned from leave in the UK after a very long tour of duty. I had heard a lot about him during his absence. For several years he had managed the farms and experimental livestock improvement projects and was very much a part of Mpwapwa. He had gone on leave as a confirmed bachelor and on his return he proudly announced that he was engaged to be married to a girl from the Isle of Man. Everybody was delighted. A young, newly recruited Veterinary Officer, Ken Aspinall, from the UK had been posted to the lab to help me while he found his sea legs before taking over a hefty rinderpest immunisation campaign in Southern Masailand. His misguided anticipation of a reasonable lifestyle in His Majesty's Colonial Service evaporated when he learnt that he, loads and all, was to share the tiny rest house with me. However, not long thereafter, a fine house next to CJ's own, overlooking the golf course, became vacant and we both moved in.

Another attraction of the move was that CJ, being an old-timer, had a short wave radio which we made frequent use of in following the exciting news leading up to the cessation of hostilities in Europe.

More immediate excitement was the news that His Excellency the Governor (actually an Acting Governor, pending the arrival of the substantive official), accompanied by his wife, was to pay an official visit to Mpwapwa. At that time the Empire was still very much up and running and the Governor as the Viceroy of H.M. King George VI was accorded due respect. As well, the fortunes of the Department depended to a large extent on his being kept aware of the importance of its work and the efficiency of its management. I was told in no uncertain terms that I had a week to see that the lab, its facilities and its personnel were spick and span. A team of labourers headed by one of the Apprentice Stock Inspectors soon had the laboratory building and even the curb stones leading up to the entrance sparkling in fresh whitewash. The animal buildings were whitewashed inside and out with not a wisp of hay out of place. The Zoo was spring-cleaned and the warthog's hooves checked for excessive growth. The lab furniture, instruments and even the buttons of the uniformed staff were burnished bright. The lab assistants were warned to have freshly laundered white coats ready for the day. Arrangements were made for a bunch of our biggest draft oxen to be ready in the entrance pen of the cattle dip so that His Excellency could enjoy the impressive spectacle of these hefty beasts launching themselves off the end of the entrance race and taking the plunge with a great splash.

On the appointed morning the Governor's special train arrived at Gulwe Station where the Director of Veterinary Services and the local District Officer were waiting. The official limousine was off-loaded, the flag fixed in place on the bonnet and the rather incongruous little procession set off along the dirt road to Mpwapwa throwing up clouds of dust. The rains had petered out about two weeks previously, so dust was once more the order of the day. As the cars approached the village of Mpwapwa little groups of terrified women on their way to the market must have been scattered, characteristically losing their head loads in the process, as this bizarre cavalcade took them by surprise coming round the corners.

The first stop was at the laboratory where I was waiting at the entrance to the veranda dressed in collar and tie, long trousers and clean

white coat, to receive the party. I did so with trepidation, despite memories of my relaxed chat with His Grace the Duke of Devonshire only
several months previously. The Director and I took turns on the conducted tour of the various laboratories, library, rinderpest *boma*, guinea
pigs, rabbits and so on, introducing as many members of staff as possible.
Sadly, our initial enthusiastic commentaries drifted into rather dull, stupid-
sounding monologues like one of those speeches that have gone wrong
when you can hear your own detached voice coming from somewhere a
few feet above your head. Even the zoo, which I had kept up my sleeve
as a prelude to the grand finale - the cattle dip - seemed hardly worth visiting. The mood had become such that the spectacular plunge of the great
oxen into the dip tank elicited little more from the assembled party than
the nodding of a few heads. After a tour of the farms a small group was
entertained to lunch at the Director's house. The Director as the senior
official was seated on the right of the Governor's wife. The senior lady
on the station, Peggy Holloway, (the wife of a Livestock Officer, Jack
Holloway, whose work took him away from Mpwapwa on long safaris
throughout the year) had supervised the preparation of the excellent meal
and was seated on the Governor's left while I was on his right. I was
intrigued to find that protocol ordained that His Excellency as the first in
the land was served first but I was even more surprised when he immediately set to with gusto before the waiter even got down to his wife.
Apparently, this was the accepted procedure for kings and viceroys. It all
rolled off my friend Ken, a blunt straight-speaking native of Blackpool,
who stretched out for the butter dish and reached it just an inch ahead of
the Governor. After a split second's hesitation Ken helped himself to a
portion and immediately passed it back to His Excellency with a knowing smile, as if to say "gotcha"!

The V.E. celebrations were much more fun. It had been obvious for
some time that the war in Europe was almost over and by Monday 7 May
the official news was expected at any moment. I was instructed to wait
on at the lab for a phone call from Head Office confirming that Europe
was officially at peace, whereupon I was to blow the siren. By 6 p.m. no
word had come through so all of the Europeans present in Mpwapwa at
the time (twelve men, four wives and a few children home from school
in Kenya) gathered at Neil and Gwen Reid's house to listen to the radio.

Eventually, at 9 p.m. we heard that the war was over. It was a momentous occasion, marked by a kaleidoscope of conflicting emotions ranging from excitement, bearing on almost uncontrollable hilarity, through to a great sense of relief, mixed with deep sorrow at the memory of loved ones and friends who had been killed or maimed during the past five years. Even though Tanganyika had escaped the actual hostilities few present that night had completely escaped the tragedies and deprivations of war. Among the company were two Italian prisoners of war who had been confined to Mpwapwa, more or less as ticket-of-leave men, since the defeat of the Italian forces in Ethiopia. There had never been any risk of their escaping because there was simply no place for them to go. In any case they had become well liked members of the community, who were respected for their competence as mechanical engineers in keeping the Department's ageing vehicles, other machinery and equipment in service with the minimum of facilities. When they did not have the necessary tools they just got down and made them. Their joy that night at the prospect of being united at long last with their families in their beloved Italy was infectious.

Mention of the Italians brings to mind the Polish people who, when caught between the advancing German and Russian armies in the early stages of the war, had opted to flee southwards by whatever means possible. More than 5,000 of them had somehow managed to reach Tanganyika and had been living since then in great boredom in crowded refugee camps in certain parts of the country.

However, it was above all a time for rejoicing so Neil Reid set off through the darkness to the CMS Mission a few miles out in bush to borrow a little portable organ. That was the best we could do for music. As soon as it was assembled Peggy Holloway, who had a lovely voice with which she entertained us at all the parties, started the ball rolling. That was followed by a singsong largely of Scottish and Irish songs interspersed with a few touching Italian tenor solos. What a feeble celebration it would have seemed to those huge congregations of people who were rolling out the barrel in more populous parts of the world. Nevertheless, our simple commemoration behind the few lighted windows in the pitch dark loneliness of the Kikombo valley had a quality of its own.

Next day, Tuesday 8 May, was designated V.E. Day, a public holiday for celebrations throughout the country. First job was up to the laboratory to slaughter seven bullocks for meat to distribute that afternoon to the African staff and labourers for their celebrations. By 10 a.m. all of the staff from the laboratory, farms and Head Office were on their way down to Mpwapwa Village attired in their best clothes for the official celebration of the formal surrender of the German forces to the Allies. The veterinary trucks and such cars as we had were gaily decorated with flowers and flags and were otherwise crammed to capacity by all those who had managed to scramble aboard. In the village we were joined by the party from the Mpwapwa Secondary School, one of the few secondary schools in the country. It was led by the school's band followed by the scholars. Behind them came the school's equally well decorated lorry with the Principal, Mr Blumer, and his wife, the African teachers and the Australian missionary on board followed by the veterinary vehicles. The rear was brought up by the bulk of the general populace of Mpwapa.

Cheering children and keening African ladies colourfully attired in *kitambas* skipped alongside the whole procession. The keen was an exciting, high-pitched, ululation produced by wagging the outstretched tongue against the open lips. *Kitambas* are brightly coloured tablecloth-like cotton sheets hitched around their bodies from the knees to the shoulders and knotted around the neck, many of them, on this occasion, bearing brilliant legends such as 'God Save the King' stretched across the ample bottoms of the older ladies.

The procession made its way to the school's football field where one of the trucks was cleared to make room for Neil Reid (in the absence of the Director who was off on safari), the District Officer, Mr Blumer and the Missionary to conduct the ceremonies. The District Officer announced that the war in Europe was over and called for three thundering cheers. The Missionary offered a prayer of thanksgiving. Then Mr Blumer called on the School choir to lead the singing. Finally, Neil was rewarded with what is best described as the father and mother of a standing ovation when he announced that seven oxen had been slaughtered. The meat was to be distributed for feasting that night.

After the formalities on the football field the assembled crowd broke up and continued the celebrations that night in their own particular ethnic groups. The whites from the Veterinary Department and those from the school and the District Office down in Mpwapwa village gathered together in the library at the laboratory where a few carpets had been laid down. We had all raided our 'peace stores' so there was plenty to drink and the ladies had laid on a memorable spread that included long-forgotten delicacies. But before the festivities began the centrepiece was the Reid's short wave radio wired up to a 12-volt car battery on which we heard a service of thanksgiving and the King's speech. Once again, I suppose our feelings of relief and pleasure in anticipating all the good things (such as closer contact with families at home, cars, radios, fridges, and home leave) that peace would bring were tinged with a sense of loneliness and sadness varying in degree from individual to individual. It became known that 8 May was my twenty-fourth birthday so after the 'Happy Birthday' chorus I had to do my party piece.

We had two visitors in our company that night; an elderly retired Medical Officer and his wife. The doctor had leprosy, which in those days was untreatable, and he was either discouraged from settling back home in England, or disinclined to do so, when sea passages became available. Their sorrow was two-fold, as he quietly confided to me later that night. His only son's birthday coincided with mine - he would have been twenty-five that very day - but all the poor couple had to look forward to was receiving the Victoria Cross that had recently been awarded to their son posthumously for bravery in Burma. It was probably the first time I had learnt how impossible it is to realise the depth of unhappiness that too often lies behind a seemingly tranquil face.

The benefits of peace began to appear remarkably soon after VE Day, even though the war in the Far East still raged on. Almost immediately, censorship of communications between Great Britain and Ireland and, presumably, many other countries was lifted and before long letters began to arrive from Ireland and the U.K. devoid of the familiar OPENED BY CENSOR label. It was a particularly happy day when my mail contained the first copy of the Irish Times that I had seen since leaving home, still printed on the distinctly off-white, wartime newsprint.

The last rains had fallen shortly before VE Day so the dry season was now well established. The damage done to the earth roads during the rains had been repaired by filling in patches that had been washed away, mending broken culverts and making the whole road up with fresh laterite dug out of holes along the roadside. Railway embankments where wash-aways had seriously damaged the 'permanent way' and closed the line from Dar for days on end on several occasions during the rains were more thoroughly repaired. Labour for the roads was supplied by the local chiefs throughout the whole country as a matter of course and the work was conducted without hassle under the immediate supervision of a head-man from the nearest village and the watchful eye of the local District Officers. It was a seasonal chore that we all noticed with pleasure in passing as marking the beginning of another dry season and easier travel after the difficulty of getting about and the feeling of confinement during the rains. The mending of the roads was followed by a general increase in movement throughout the whole country and visits to remote places, which might have been impossible during the wet season, were now undertaken.

Mpwawa had its full share of seasonal visitors that year. The first to arrive was the new Governor who stopped off at Mpwapwa during an extensive tour up-country. The preparations were just as thorough but much easier as a repeat performance. His Excellency was most receptive and seemed keenly interested in all that was going on.

The next visitor was an elderly professor of entomology from the U.K. His visit followed the receipt by me, from an unknown source, of no less than a barrel of the new wonder insecticide DDT. It had been unaccompanied by any information as to how it might be used so it was good to meet the professor who was an authority on the subject. He had flown out to East Africa to check out centres where basic facilities might be developed for investigating how DDT might be used for the control of certain diseases of man and animals transmitted by insects and other arthropods.

In appearance he was a caricature of the absent-minded professor. Nevertheless, he knew exactly what he was after and went through a long list of searching questions as to what the laboratory had to offer. He was short on small talk so it was a relief when he asked to borrow a rucksack so that he could search for some riverine insects. I escorted him to a little stream bubbling out of thick bush on the side of a nearby hill. Just as he disappeared into bush with his long-shafted butterfly net he spotted an Acacia tree displaying a spectacular array of yellow flowers and, despite his difficulty with small talk, he turned and exclaimed: 'A pleasant plant, a showy shrub, a member of the Acacia family I venture. Aye, a handsome bloom'. At a loss for a suitable reply, I pleaded my need to return to the lab.

In retrospect, I marvel at the naivety of people like myself and even distinguished scientists of those days who heralded the arrival of the synthetic chlorinated hydrocarbon insecticides as panaceas for the control or even, in some circumstances, the eradication of some of the most troublesome diseases of man and animals in the tropics, such as malaria, trypanosomiasis (sleeping sickness of man and other manifestations of the disease in animals) and a whole variety of tick-borne diseases. Even the unselective activity of DDT and its long residual effects were received with acclaim. For many years, few seemed to appreciate the potential dangers of, for example, spraying huge tracts of tsetse bush with broad spectrum insecticides that killed not only the tsetse fly but also a wide variety of other species of arthropods that play a vital role in the ecology of any given area. The additional dangers of using a non-degradable chemical for such purposes was also ignored initially, as was the ease with which such substances can enter and accumulate in the food chain of animals.

The next important visitation was a conference of Provincial Veterinary Officers from each of the seven provinces. Normally, the co-ordination of the provincial activities was effected by the Director or Neil Reid, the Senior Veterinary Officer at Headquarters, travelling around the huge Territory on safari. The Conference brought together all of the PVOs and the Headquarters staff, including our new Pasture Research Officer, Van Rensburg, and myself. That left only a handful of the more junior Veterinary Officers in the field, either temporarily in charge of a province or out in bush running immunisation camps. Transmissible diseases recognise no boundaries, nor do pastoral people, such as the Masai. As well, the system of stock routes operated by the Department, like the route running for hundreds of miles from Western Province through the Lake and Northern Provinces to Nairobi in Kenya, provide an excellent conduit for the passage of disease. The ending of the war in Europe also provided a greater incentive to plan for the future. The Conference enabled such matters to be discussed collectively.

For me personally, it was exciting meeting, face to face, members of the staff from whom I had been receiving diagnostic material. As well, any one of them might well become my next boss because word had got round that Jack Wilde was expected back from leave in two months time whereupon I would be posted to the field. The PVOs were desperate for staff so I found myself in a happy position as a scarce commodity. Some surreptitious conversations took place and the best offer came, perhaps not surprisingly, from an Irishman Mike Molloy, who was a Senior Veterinary Officer for whom I had diagnosed tuberculosis in poultry and tried to type the bovine strain of the tubercule from cattle. Tuberculosis in cattle was rearing its ugly head to a serious extent in his Province. One offer was Iringa District only a hundred and fifty miles south of Mpwapwa in the cool of his beautiful Southern Highlands Province. Amongst other attractions, he was building a small diagnostic lab there and already had a laboratory technician. What more could I wish for - the rest was up to him. He raised the problem of bovine tuberculosis in the Southern Highlands on every possible occasion during the Conference and reported back to me that he had had a word with Neil Reid who was very well-disposed to the proposition. Our little intrigue came to nothing when word came through that Jack Wilde would not be returning until January, by which time I would be a year in Mpwapwa. That suited me equally well.

During the Conference I met David White and his wife Pat for the first time. David was a tall, slim man in his early thirties from the Isle of Man who had qualified in both veterinary medicine and agriculture at Edinburgh in 1939 just before the outbreak of war. Pat was a good-looking brunette, rather younger and smaller in stature than her husband but every bit as kind and big-hearted as he was. David had recently been appointed P.V.O. of Central Province of which Mpwapwa District was a part. They were stationed at Dodoma, the Provincial Headquarters only seventy miles away. It was the beginning of a warm friendship which, amongst other things, gave me and some of my bachelor friends at Mpwapwa access to an open door and a bed on the veranda at Dodoma, as well as invitations to dances at the Club where the chances of meeting an unattached girl increased gradually from absolute zero to 1 in 1000 as more passages from the U.K. began to offer a few opportunities for younger sisters to visit their relatives. In the absence of female company, the

Mpwapwa bachelors were spoilt by Pat with her access to the gradually increasing supply of consumer goods coming on to the shelves of the Indian *dukas* in Dodoma. On one of Pat's subsequent visits I found, to my great surprise, that she had transformed my bachelor abode. When I walked in from the lab the sitting room was brilliant. Floral curtains draped the windows instead of the flat unpleated purple hessian and matching covers concealed the khaki cushions of the Public Works Department's armchairs. The measurements had been taken surreptitiously on Pat's previous visit.

By the time the Japanese cabinet decided to surrender on 10 August another mini-war had broken out at Mpwapwa. The aggressor was a lion. During the dry season watering points dried up on the semi-arid plains surrounding the Kiboriana Mountains and game scattered. Lions tended to retreat into the foothills that sweep down to our cleared valleys. Some game animals followed suit but our cattle, which grazed under the care of herdsmen by day and were confined in *bomas* by night, were easier prey. My first experience was an attack during the early hours of the morning on an outlying cattle *boma* up the valley. It was a large circular enclosure, capable of holding about a hundred head of cattle, with a strong perimeter fence about nine to ten feet high made of relatively straight bush poles. The herd boys in a nearby hut had heard the commotion but were too scared to go out. At one point there was a ragged bloodstained patch where the lion had either heaved or tossed a bullock over the top of the fence. Outside, we found a trail that led to the kill a few hundreds yards away but there was no sign of the lion. It shocked me to see for the first time evidence of the frightening strength of a lion. It filled me with a healthy respect. This was no hand fed zoo animal safely confined behind bars - it was a wild beast that at any time might well emerge from the long grass as one walked or rode the horses through the relatively confined Kikombo valley.

There was still plenty of the carcass left so Phillip Princello and I borrowed the staff car and returned that night shortly after sunset; we parked at a respectful distance from the kill. There was some moonlight that night and being in the safety of the staff car there was no need for both of us to keep our eyes skinned on the kill so we agreed to take turns at dozing off for an hour at a time. At about 4 a.m., as it subsequently transpired, I got a nudge and a whisper from Phillip. I was immediately wide awake and held my breath with excitement as I perceived the outline of my first lion settling down at the kill. Phillip, the son of Boers who had settled in East Africa, had hunting in his blood and practical experience since his childhood. So, as the lion was obviously oblivious of our presence, we sat quietly for a few moments while Phillip explained his strategy in whispers. Then he gently eased his door wide open, slipped out with rifle in hand and crept forward a little in order to get a better view of his sights when I switched on the car lights. At a pre-arranged signal from Phillip I switched on the headlights. Almost simultaneously, the rifle cracked and, sadly, cracked again as the lion bounded off in the full glare of the headlights towards a bush-clad hillside. Though it was disappointing for Phillip, I was well satisfied to see my first lion in the wild and to have it impressed on me by the chirping of the cicadas and other night noises that this was it - not a zoo job. Next day there was no sign of the carcass, not even a bone or a piece of hide, but it was later found in the bush about a quarter of a mile away.

During the next three weeks, a cow, two more bullocks and a donkey were taken and there was not much we could do other than strengthen the walls of the outlying *boma*s with surrounds of thorn bush. Everybody, blacks and whites, were conscious that a lion was abroad so there was no longer any question of walking outdoors after dark, other than to nip across to a nearby house and we were wary on our daylight leisure pursuits after work, such as horse riding or shooting.

Despite our respect for the lion, Phillip and I were misguidedly prompted by the impetuousness of youth to attempt to confront him at Nunge Dairy where he had killed a cow in unusual circumstances. Nunge, which was located about a mile from the laboratory, was a conventional European-type farmyard with corrugated iron-roofed cowshed which housed the cows for milking and during the night. Each animal, including the bull, was tethered in an individual stall by means of a neck chain attached to a stanchion. Near one end of the cowshed proper there was a two roomed mud hut that served as a sickbay. On the night of the raid there was a cow in one of the rooms, so to gain access the lion had jumped on to the roof and torn a hole through the thatch near the middle of the ridge. This gave it ample access to the cow's compartment though there was also a small opening into the adjoining room which was separated from the other by a lattice-work partition made from bush poles. The lion had dropped down on to the unfortunate cow and presumably dispatched her immediately. Having had his fill, he must have made his exit by leaping up through the hole in the roof because the door into the cow's compartment remained intact.

In anticipation of his coming back for another feed on the following night, Phillip and I returned before sunset with my motorbike and took up our position in the empty compartment. It had seemed a good idea earlier in the day but as we faced the reality of the approaching darkness the partition between us and the carcass looked uncomfortably fragile. The hole in the roof on our side of the partition was also more threatening. We did, at least, have the good sense to leave the door into the cow's compartment open to encourage the lion to come in that way rather than dropping down on us from the hole in the roof. In any event, the strategy was to settle down for the night on a comfortable bed of straw in the empty compartment, one on either side of the motorbike. The latter would be propped up between us with the headlight pointing through the gaps in the partition at the kill. We were both armed with double barrelled shotguns loaded with (large) SSG shot for close encounter; we also had a rifle and a pistol within easy reach, just in case. As soon as the lion appeared in the doorway, the idea was to blind it with light from the motorbike's headlamp and then blast away simultaneously with four barrels of SSG. It seemed a great idea provided the lion did not drop in on top of us through the hole in the roof.

After an hour or two listening to the night noises we heard the unmistakable roar of a lion from the hills at the other side of the valley. The roar had been heard by all the other living creatures and, as happens on such occasions, it was followed by deadly silence; the lion was on his way. As the night wore on we took turns at dozing until, suddenly, we were both brought wide awake by an almighty roar from the vicinity of the nearby cow house. Nothing more happened and after a tense period of waiting we gradually relaxed and resumed our spells of dozing. Just before daybreak another roar brought both of us to action stations again, with me holding my shotgun with one hand and the other on the headlamp while Phillip was at the other side of the bike grasping his shotgun with the revolver within easy reach. This time the roar was followed by the rattle of loose corrugated iron sheets as the lion prowled along the roof of the cowshed. Could he possibly jump across the gap between the cowshed and the roof of the hut; if so, would he bring the whole roof in on top of us? We were in a dilemma. It would have been ridiculous to go out in the pitch dark to search for a lion at such short range with a flash lamp. On the other hand, it was frustrating and frightening after such a long night to be so close to the brute that had caused so much havoc. Needless to say, we temporized until there was nearly enough light to venture cautiously outside. Just as we reached the bull's stall at the far end of the shed there was an almighty roar followed immediately by more rattling on the iron roof, or so it seemed. But good grief, it was not so, it was merely the bull roaring as he rattled his chain up and down the stanchion as he greeted the arrival of the dawn!

The next major excitement began one Saturday a few weeks later. At about 10.30 p.m. I received word that two of my experimental calves had just been killed at Nunge Dairy about a quarter of a mile up the valley quite close to Willie Burns' house. I was having a drink with CJ and David White who had brought an Army officer through from Dodoma for the weekend. They had travelled in an army lorry that was fitted with a searchlight on the top of the cab. We threw a few armchairs up on the lorry and climbed aboard with rifles and double barrel shotguns. The shotguns loaded with SSG cartridges containing an extra heavy charge and only oversize lead pellets gave one great comfort at close quarters, especially after dark, when it was difficult to aim accurately with a rifle. On arrival at the scene of the crime we found that the lion had been frightened away by the brave herdsmen armed only with spears so we toured up and down the valleys in the rather vain hope of picking up the culprit in the beam of the searchlight. It was to no avail but we were surprised by the amount and variety of wildlife shown up by our new toy the searchlight, such as bush buck, duiker, dik dik, civet and serval cats and a few jackal.

Next day before breakfast I slipped up to the laboratory to do a few jobs in the quiet of a Sunday morning. I was met by an agitated attendant who greeted me with 'Ah, *tabu nyingi*, Bwana!' (much trouble). The lion had broken into the zoo and created havoc. He had actually scaled the eight-foot high brick wall and killed three bush buck and a Thompson's gazelle. At first, the number of animals wantonly killed and the scaling of the wall suggested that it was the work of a leopard because the leopard tends to kill just for the fun of it. Indeed, a leopard had scaled an identical wall of the nearby goat *boma* a couple of months previously and killed thirteen goats but had apparently carried only one away. However, spoor on some wet ground inside showed that the visitor had been a lion. In any case, the damage to the pens could not have been inflicted by a leopard. The place looked as if a bomb had hit it. In the confines of the zoo the panic must have been intense. Five pens were flattened, wooden partitions and wire were scattered everywhere, the roof of a shelter staved in and a brick wall knocked down.

It was now about 8 a.m. While we were still viewing the damage in disbelief, a herd boy who had just then taken a herd of cattle out to graze rushed in and told us that the lion had sprung out of long grass only a few hundred yards from the laboratory and brought one of the cows down. By this time Mpwapwa was astir and shocked that such a daring lion was not only loose in the valley, but also prepared to strike so close to the dwellings. A party of about eight Europeans armed to the teeth with rifles and shotguns and several Africans with spears made its way as quietly as possible to the nearby kill and arrived just in time to see the lion disappearing into a dry, bush-clad river bed running up the side of the mountain. Two of the most experienced Europeans followed it into the bush - somebody would have been shot if more had joined them. It was a perilous exercise scrambling up the bottom of the narrow watercourse because if the lion had gained the higher ground the two could have been pounced on from the dense undergrowth. They soon had the good sense to call it off.

But this could not be allowed to go on so we were forced to respond unsportingly by attempting to poison the beast. Barium chloride is now an obsolete drug that was once used in very small doses for the treatment of colic in horses. I had read about its use as bait poison so later that morning I was delighted to find some in the stores. Phillip and I managed to prepare a large quantity of a concentrated solution in water which we injected into several parts of the hump and liver of the morning's kill, using rubber gloves and a hypodermic syringe with a very long needle. It was essential not to touch the carcass with naked hands. At toxic dosage rates the drug induces powerful contractions of the entire length of the intestinal tract which soon produces violent straining and copious diarrhoea. This can go on for several hours and in terminal cases ends in heart failure. Next morning we were delighted to find that most of the liver had been eaten but disappointed that there were no signs of diarrhoea in the vicinity of the kill, nor did we ever find a lion carcass during extensive searches of the nearby bush. There were no more attacks, however, during the remainder of that dry season. That was a bit unsatisfactory as it would have been interesting to know who had won, though the uncertainty was probably fitting retribution for our unsporting behaviour in trying to dispose of the king of the beasts by a method one uses, without thinking, against common vermin.

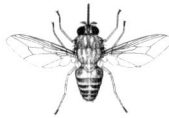

CHAPTER THIRTEEN

An Immunisation Camp
on the Masai Steppes

A welcome safari in Masailand, under canvas for the first time, to see a rinderpest immunisation campaign in action. Learning about White Hunters, shooting elephants and hearing stories of the German army in a rearguard action in East Africa during the First World War.

Nineteen forty-five had, so far, been a bad year for rinderpest. When Ian Macadam was transferred precipitately to the Singida District of Central Province, he was shocked by the sight of some five hundred carcasses covering a discrete patch of bush. This was his first experience of the disease in the field. Concurrently, there was a mild form smouldering away at Tabora on the Central Railway line which was extremely difficult to diagnose. By contrast, a very serious epizootic in cattle and game up north was spreading from Tanga Province, which borders on Kenya, westwards and southwards across the Ruvu River into Masailand. The virus involved was distinctly virulent, affecting cattle as well as a wide variety of game including impala, oryx, waterbuck and Grant's gazelle which had previously been regarded as being less susceptible than the usual carriers such as buffalo, eland, giraffe, pig and wildebeest.

In August, concern about the possibility of the mild form of the disease at Tabora slipping undetected southwards through sparsely populated country towards the Northern Rhodesian border was such that representatives of the Union of South Africa, Southern and Northern Rhodesia, Nyasaland, Portuguese East Africa, Belgian Congo, Rwanda-Urundi, Kenya, Uganda and Tanganyika met in Nairobi. Agreement was reached as to how the disease should be tackled in East Africa generally.

Earlier the Mpwapwa Conference of Provincial Veterinary Officers had already decided that an immunisation campaign extending from the Central Railway line northwards towards the Kenya border should be undertaken. Ken Aspinall was already busy inoculating all the cattle in an area measuring 150 miles by 90 miles in Southern Masailand. Other teams were engaged with outbreaks elsewhere. Adult stock was being immunised with the Kenya Dried Goat Virus that was easily transported, each small vial containing 250 doses. The cold chain required for the storage of this vaccine out in bush was reasonably easily taken care of by fridges running on paraffin which were carried hither and thither in wooden crates. Thermos flasks were used for local distribution. My robust, unsophisticated old vaccine, which was reserved for calves and yearlings, was trundled around without a care over appalling roads and across trackless country in crates of beer bottles.

The orders for the Mpwapwa vaccine began to pile up; at the end of August I was asked to produce 390 litres (39,000 doses) forthwith. This involved infecting and slaughtering fifteen bullocks every second day so that vaccine production continued uninterrupted seven days a week for three weeks. We were all jaded by the time the order was completed and at that point an SOS for vaccine and other supplies arrived from Ken Aspinall, 125 miles away at Kibaya at the southern edge of the Masai Steepe. Willie Burns, the Deputy Director at Head Office, considered I needed a break and insisted that I accompany the consignment and take a few days up there to see what went on at the consumer's end. I protested that there was far too much accumulated work to be done but, kind man that he was, he ordered me to make a list of all that needed attention. He would see that it was done in my absence. Once down on paper it did not seem so bad. Nevertheless, during the course of checking the fridges I discovered that no reserves of rinderpest-infected spleen had been laid down during the past three months. Infected spleen, in which the virus was more stable than in blood, was our fail-safe reserve stock. Had there been a break in our vaccine production with a consequent interruption in blood passages we could well have lost the vaccine strain that had been in use for the past eight years. One had always to be on the alert, constantly checking that delegated procedures were being carried out. If the virus had been lost, instead of going to Masailand I would have been heading home! I considered myself lucky that the incessant demand for more and more vaccine at the time had necessitated the passage of infective blood into fresh groups of susceptible cattle every second day of the week. In no uncertain terms it was arranged that samples of infective spleen would be in the fridge on my return.

Next morning was a bright, sunny day with thin white ribbons of cloud trailing along the side of Kiborani Mountain well clear of the peaks. I was glad to have secured the much-loved three ton ex-army lorry, affectionately nick-named the "Yellow Peril". It had seen service in the desert – hence its yellow colour – but it was still utterly reliable. It was soon loaded with crates of vaccine, drums of petrol, guns, bags of meal and rice, other provisions for Ken and, above all, a tent and camp bed for the Bwana in case we got stuck on the way. At the last minute Neil Reid arrived with four elephant tusks which we were to take on the first stage of their journey to an ivory dealer in Tanga. The sale of ivory was legal in those days, though the game licence was restricted to the shooting of two animals per year. The turney boy, a Veterinary Guard and my two chaps, along with the inevitable passengers who had heard that we were heading north, climbed aboard and we were on our way. There was no harm in having a few extra hands in case we had to dig ourselves out of the loose sand in the dry river beds which were so prevalent at that stage of the dry season. There had not been a drop of rain for the past five months. As we sped down the narrow valley to the village in the cool morning air and out into the open country, all the worries of Mpwapwa evaporated at the thought of three days of complete freedom ahead.

The shadows were shortening and the temperatures rising as we drove past cultivated stretches of Ugogo (the land of the Wagogo people on Central Province), now reddish-brown with withered stubble. It was entertaining to watch mini-tornadoes, the so-called wind devils, composed of thin columns of sand and debris being sucked high into the sky, twisting and turning across the bone dry landscape. We had been making up to thirty miles per hour over reasonably good roads but by midday we were for the most part following wheel tracks through unpopulated country, often down to five miles per hour and sometimes digging ourselves out of sand as we crossed dry river beds.

Despite the dryness of the terrain there must have been water somewhere because there was now plenty of game, including large herds of

Thompson's gazelle, Grant's gazelle, zebra, giraffe, and there was even elephant dung. The game grazed contentedly within easy range of us and were obviously untroubled by man. On the other hand, the warthogs which we encountered from time to time scurried away with rigid tails sticking vertically upwards like radio antennae, somewhat reminiscent of the frigates I had seen fussing around the convoy as we assembled in the mouth of the Mersey almost a year ago. What a contrast between that cold, grey, hostile seascape and this bright, warm, seemingly peaceful landscape which must have here remained largely undisturbed by human intervention through countless years. On the other hand, some of the game we passed were the very species which probably facilitated the southward passage of rinderpest that at the turn of the century practically wiped out the Masai herds, and indeed the Masai themselves because of their dependence on cattle rather than arable farming for their sustenance. The heat of the afternoon sun and the steady drone of the Yellow Peril's engine induced a somnolence that was conducive to inconsequential, philosophical reverie.

We arrived out of the darkness at the immunisation camp near Kibaya, wherever or whatever that was, to take Ken Aspinall and his companion, Basil Reel, completely by surprise. Ken was at the back of his tent with legs hanging out over the edge of his shiny, new, all-purpose, portable safari bath not long off the shelves of Griffiths McAlister, London. With a shout of delight he hobbled around, clutching a towel despite the cold that was now descending, to greet us at the front of the tent where a campfire was burning merrily. Basil Reel was introduced and cold beer was extracted from between boxes of KAG vaccine in the portable fridge. We settled down around the fire as we were - Ken had no thought of dressing for dinner, with or without a black tie; the beer and the need to talk to a stranger was too pressing. My travelling companions, who had been warmly welcomed with many cries of '*habari ya safari's?*' (how was the safari?) and much shaking of hands, were now settling around their own fire where the resident cook was already cooking dinner. There was not much to the camp other than Ken's and Basil's tents, another couple of tents and a few huts that served as accommodation for the veterinary and domestic staff and stores.

After an excellent meal our fire was made up before we retired to bed by one of the boys who then settled down beside it and kept it fuelled during the night as a precaution against lions and other predators. This was my first night out in bush. As I lay in my brand new camp bed after everything had settled down, I was fascinated by the constant background night noise of the cicadas punctuated by the barking of jackals and the eerie two-toned cry of hyaenas, not all that far off.

Next morning, after a breakfast of fried egg, with much-appreciated bacon and sausage straight from Bwana Bain's, Ken was itching to take me on what proved to be a long tour to see more game and some of the other camps where he had been inoculating within his 150 by 90 mile block. The first stop was at the home cattle crush which was only a few hundred yards from the tents. It was already in full swing.

The crush consisted of a narrow passage with sides about five feet high made from stout bush poles driven securely into the ground and bound tightly together with sisal or bark rope. The actual crush was about fifty yards long; it was important that it should be narrow enough to prevent cattle turning around while they were being packed in. There was nothing worse than to have an animal struggling around to squeeze past the one behind, thereby creating an almost inextricable logjam. It was essential to ensure that the walls were high enough to prevent the larger bullocks jumping out so an earthen bank was thrown up along one side of the passage to give the inoculators sufficient height from which to lean down into the crush when injecting the vaccine. At one end there was a holding enclosure or *boma* to accommodate the herd entering the crush and another at the far end in which the herd being injected assembled before being driven home. Once the long line of animals was confined in the crush, the actual inoculations were performed at remarkable speed. There were three inoculators, each with his syringe and bowl of vaccine, attending to the section of the crush allotted to him. Each inoculator was served by a brander who rushed from a nearby fire with a hot branding iron and seared the letter "R" on to the backside of the cattle almost as soon as they had been injected. The operation of getting a herd into the holding pen, cramming as many cattle as possible into the crush, the darting of the inoculators and branders up and down the crush, the noisy altercations, banter and laughter of operatives and herdsmen, and the bellowing of the cattle, all created a scene of boisterous activity. Despite the noise it was a remarkably efficient undertaking whereby three to five thousand cattle could be dealt with per day, provided the herds kept coming in. It was essentially a production line, made entirely from local materials, the like of which could not have been bettered by Henry Ford when he set up his first system for the assembly of his Model T Fords.

The phased arrival of the herds was facilitated by Veterinary Guards visiting the surrounding Masai villages and assigning the days on which the different herds were to be driven to the immunisation camp. As we stood at the crush we could see several columns of dust on the horizon marking the location of herds making their way to the camp. There was little or no difficulty in persuading each village to bring their herds on the appointed day because of the respect that existed between the Masai and the vets based on their shared knowledge and mutual concern for cattle. Nevertheless, care was taken to ensure that there were no misunderstandings. This was effected by uniformed Rinderpest Scouts visiting each village to see that the whole herd was on its way.

After an enjoyable day bumping around Masailand I left Ken at one of his outlying camps. When I arrived back at the base camp after sundown a delightful hot bath was immediately poured for me at the back of the tent. It was wonderful how the boys managed to provide such luxuries and excellent dinners as a matter of course with the minimum of facilities, out there at the back of beyond, miles and miles from anything even resembling civilisation. There was, of course, plenty of game meat, guineafowl, and fresh cows' milk to be had daily, and when relatively perishable vegetables such as potatoes ran out there was always plenty of onions, rice and corn to fall back on. Even in the most remote areas such as this the cook managed to produce freshly cooked yeast bread every morning.

Sitting over the fire that night I was entertained to wonderful stories about Africa by Basil Reel. He had been a well known white hunter for many years before the war when the tourist trade was, to a large extent, confined to wealthy Americans who were determined to get as many trophies as possible to impress their friends back home. He was much sought after as an outstanding hunter who could provide for their comfort in bush and take them up as close as possible to prize specimens, under the protection of his unerring shot. When the war broke out Basil, along with several other white hunters in Tanganyika, was recruited into the Veterinary Department to monitor the movement of game in areas where rinderpest was either active or likely to become so. They were self-sufficient, spending practically all of their time in bush, isolated for long periods from European company. Ken was fortunate to have had Basil allocated to his unit. As a new recruit, he was taught by Basil how to live comfortably in bush and, of course, how to hunt. All of this, for which wealthy Americans had previously paid big money, was available to Ken free-of-charge at His Majesty's expense.

As a young impecunious Veterinary Officer Ken found himself in a position to augment his salary by elephant shooting. In those days, one could purchase an annual permit for £50 that allowed one to shoot two elephants within the twelve months. To get the best possible return on the investment it was necessary to find a really big bull with two good tusks. By the time I visited Kibaya, Basil had already initiated Ken in the art. To begin with, they had stalked some herds for practice, keeping down-wind to get in terrifyingly close. Eventually, word came in that there was a big tusker not too far away. They set out on foot and when they reached the spot and got within sight of the bull Basil was satisfied that this was the one they had been waiting for. They crept quietly in and, according to Ken, they got so close that they could hear the animal's bowels rumbling. At a nod from Basil, who was standing nearby with the second elephant gun at the ready, Ken raised his and fired at the pre-arranged spot. It was breathtakingly exciting but Ken admitted that after the excitement abated it was sad to see the huge creature lying there, life-less and limp.

During his story-telling Basil Reel had mentioned in passing that a lot of the fighting between the British and the Germans during the East African Campaign of 1914 to 1917 had swept down through this general area. Next day on my return journey to Mpwapwa, sitting idle in the hot cab beside the driver, the drone of the engine brought on another of my reveries. I remembered that soon after my arrival at Mpwapwa I was surprised that while we had three horses at Mpwapwa there were fewer than two hundred in the whole country. I had queried this with Willie Burns who explained that it was practically impossible to keep horses or mules in Tanganyika because of the prevalence of trypanosomiasis and African horse sickness. This had caused great difficulty to the British forces during the First World War. I subsequently got my hands on the official records of veterinary activities during the fighting in this part of the former German East Africa through which I had been travelling. The records contained an interesting reference to what amounted to the use of a primitive form of germ warfare by the German forces. According to these records, the German Commander in Chief, von Lettow-Vorbeck, used his veterinary officers to survey the country to the south during the course of his rearguard action. The surveys revealed the routes which were 'the most deadly to animal life' and these were the ones invariably chosen. He then sent strong forces of infantry to occupy positions considered most dangerous for animals and there they remained until the British mounted troops were attracted.

For example, during his retreat in 1916 from Korogue in the north to Morogoro down south on the Central Railway line, von Lettow selected a line of retreat precisely for this purpose. Incidentally, that line ran more or less parallel to, and east of, the route I was now following on my way back to Mpwapwa only thirty years later. He was followed into the trap by a British mounted brigade with artillery and animal transport. The success of his tactics can be gauged by the fact that between August and October 1916, out of a total of 14,000 horses and mules that passed along that route, 12,000 died. The figures for the whole of the campaign from 1914 to 1917 are even more horrifying. In brief, of 31,000 horses, 33,000 mules and 34,000 donkeys used by the British forces during the period 1914 to 1917 only 827, 897 and 1,402 respectively survived. It is probable that the majority died of trypanosomiasis and African horse sickness though, no doubt, poor nutrition also took its toll. Where draught oxen were used for the transport of materiel many must have been lost as a result of having trekked through extensive, innocent-looking tracts of land infested with the tick that transmits East Coast fever.

At the end of 1917 von Lettow-Vorbeck retreated from German East Africa across the River Ruvuma and penetrated deep into Portuguese East Africa (now Mozambique). By then he was out of ammunition, had no mounted troops or draught animals and so was solely dependent on his remaining porters for transport. He was pursued by British forces through Portuguese territory for another year during which time he eventually swung north and once more crossed the Ruvuma into German East Africa. During this period he continued to entice his pursuers into tsetse bush in which 'a rapid and malignant type of trypanosomiasis rendered pursuit by mounted troops impossible'. He eventually made his way to Njombe some 150 miles north of the Portuguese border near the top of Lake Nyassa and from there into Northern Rhodesia where he eventually surrendered at Abercorn (now Mbala) in Northern Rhodesia on 25 November 1918, a whole week after the cessation of hostilities in Europe. He was never defeated and was greatly admired by the opposing forces he had managed to evade with such tenacity for so long.

The statistics quoted above serve to illustrate how hostile the environment of Tanganyika was to the development of animal industry in particular and to the economy of the country at large. Even in the second half of the twentieth century, there were still exciting diseases in Europe, such as brucellosis and bovine tuberculosis, in the process of being controlled and much research to be done, but in Tanganyika the prevalence of so many highly fatal diseases was quite extraordinary in comparison. Transmissible diseases, such as trypanosomiasis and East Coast fever, closed up vast areas of the country in which it was either quite impossible or extremely difficult to keep domestic animals. Even in the established livestock areas there was no shortage of other lethal diseases. This situation was intensely stimulating to me, the young veterinarian, but at times rather too much for a few of the old salts, as I experienced on my return to Mpwapwa from Kibaya.

I arrived back at Mpwapwa after dark. Next morning while shaving I was interrupted by a very worried Willie Burns. A hundred and fifty rinderpest susceptible cattle for vaccine production had arrived the previous day and several were seriously ill. They had been trekked down from an area about sixty miles south of where Ken was busy establishing his 150 mile wide barrier of immune cattle between the tsetse belts to the east and the west. Willie was worried that this mob had possibly assisted the disease to leapfrog from Ken's area southwards almost to the railway line. We dropped everything to examine the sick cattle and then isolate the herd as best we could. We took lots of blood slides and I was relieved to find trypanosomes in the smears of nearly all the affected animals, but Willie was by no means satisfied. He was determined to satisfy himself that the basic condition was not rinderpest merely complicated by latent trypanosomiasis so we agreed that I should set up cross-immunity tests to establish that rinderpest was not involved. This involved injecting a group of five rinderpest susceptible cattle and another group of immune cattle with blood from the sick animals. The test animals were all temperatured and examined for symptoms of rinderpest daily for several days. As no symptoms developed in either group we felt justified in concluding that rinderpest was not involved.

By then the in-tray and other jobs had piled up but before long the decks were cleared and there was plenty of time in the afternoons for tennis with my good friends CJ (the Farm Manager), Van Rensburg (the Pasture Research Officer), Ray (the Head Office Executive Officer), and, from time to time, Neil Reid, the Director and Dr Dikshit (an Indian doctor in charge of the village clinic). My pal Phillip had been transferred to join Mac in Musoma District hundreds of miles away up on the Kenya border at the side of Lake Victoria. I missed his company as we used to ride out together along the trails in the cool of the evening through the valleys in the hope of shooting a few guineafowl for the pot.

On one memorable occasion we had gone further afield towards the lake at Kimogai where we knew there were lots of guineafowl. After tethering the horses we came upon an unusually large flock that was moving slowly ahead of us quite unaware of our presence as they concentrated on their feeding. I stayed where I was while Phillip sneaked off to the left through rather thicker bush to get in front of them in the hope of beating them back to me before they took flight. The little strategy worked in that they turned around and took off in my direction. It was a lovely shot and for once I beat Phillip by getting a brace with a left and a right. Unfortunately, there was a price to be paid; he too had blasted away as they took off and got me with two pellets just above the eye! We called it a day and trotted off to Dr Dikshit's surgery back at Mpwapwa. After the conventional, 'Oh my goodness!' he gave me a local anaesthetic before poking with an artery forceps into one of the spots which had been oozing a little blood. He repeated the process at another spot and after a perceptible tug he held the forceps up to show me the pellet he had just removed and exclaimed, 'Ah yes, very good you see - none of the balls have entered the brain, the skull only!' He was not only a good all-round doctor with a particular liking for surgery, he was also a competent photographer and used the latter skills to record some of his more

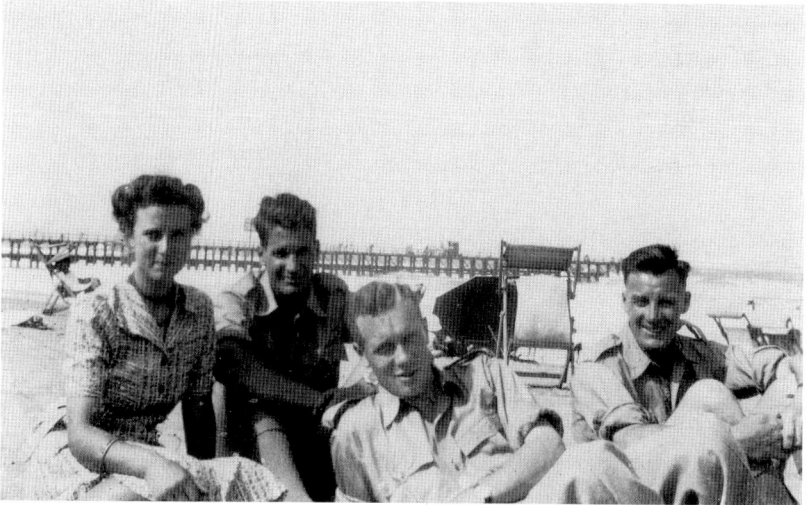

(Above) On the beach at Durban, December 1944, en route to Tanganyika: LtoR: Jean Thomas RN, Gwynn Watkins, Author, Jack Fulbeck.

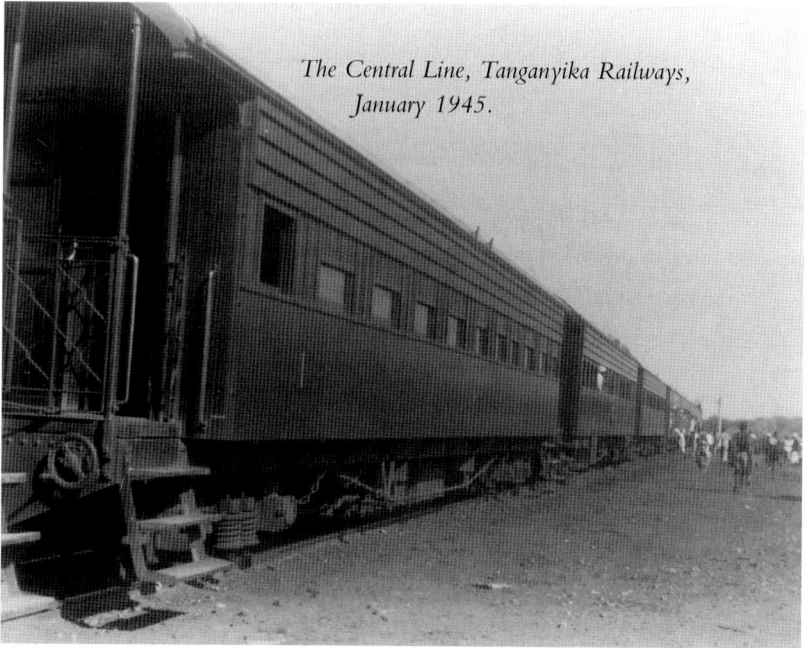

The Central Line, Tanganyika Railways, January 1945.

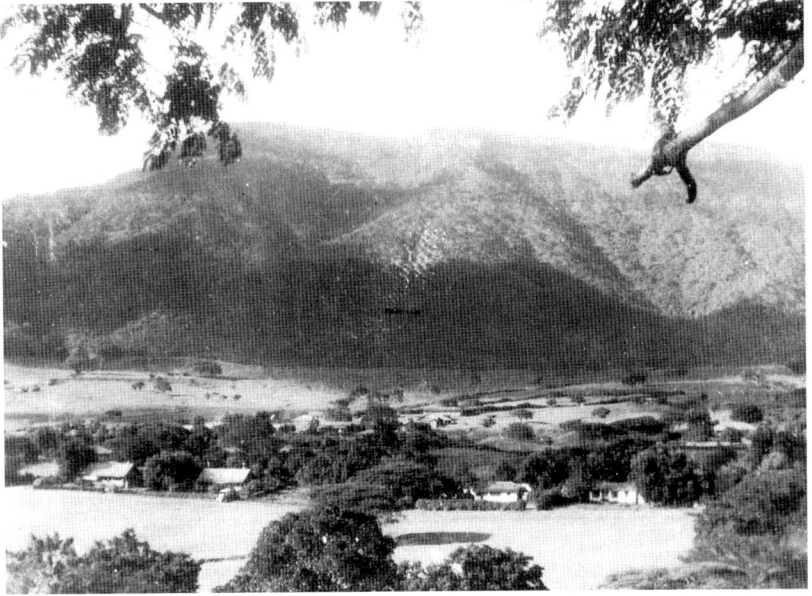

(Above) Site of the Veterinary Laboratory at Kikombo, Mpapwa with Kiboriana Mountain in background. Golf Course in foreground.

(Below) The combined staff, including Huseni, Banda, and Selemani; at back, Mac and the author.

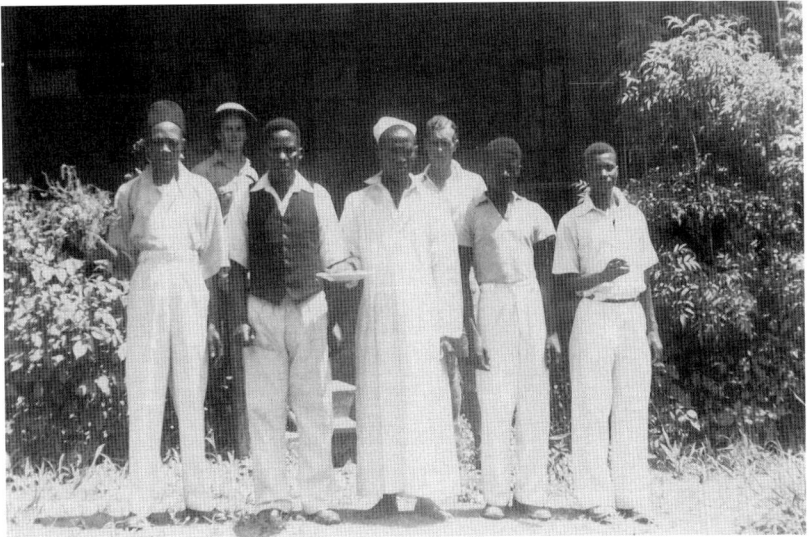

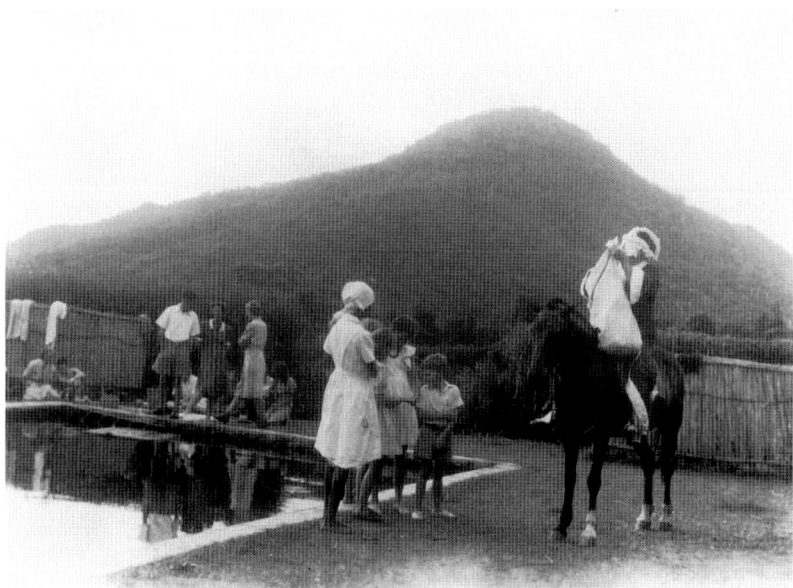

(Above) The "Irrigation Tank" at Mpwapwa.

(Below) The Veterinary Laboratory, Mpapwa 1945.

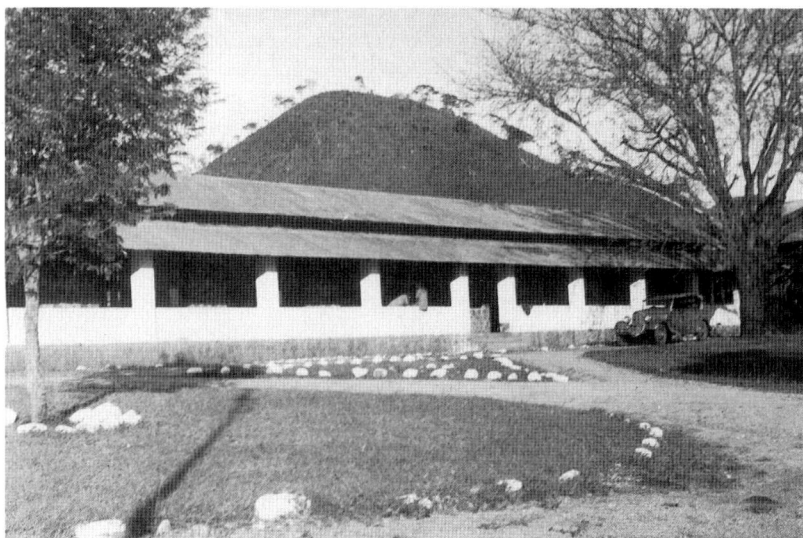

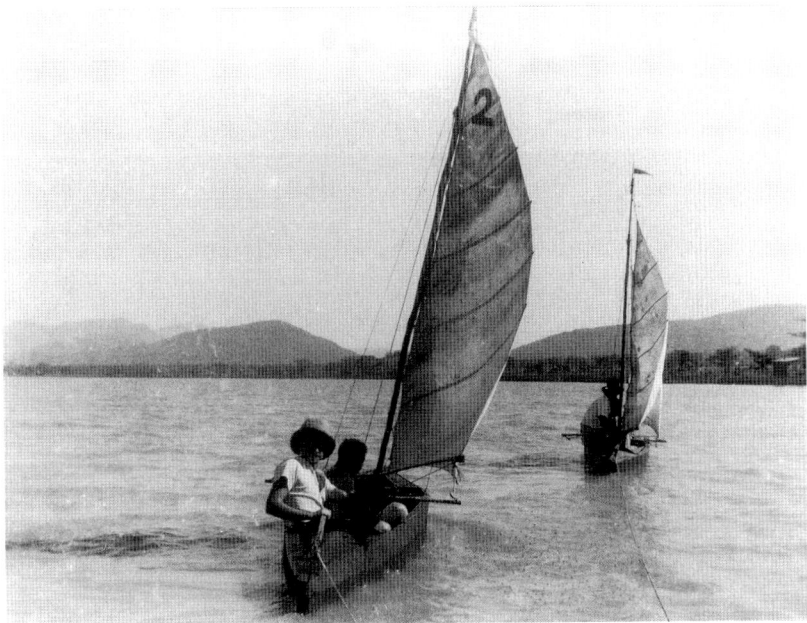

(Above) Homemade dinghies on Lake Kimagai.

(Below) Disposal of carcases

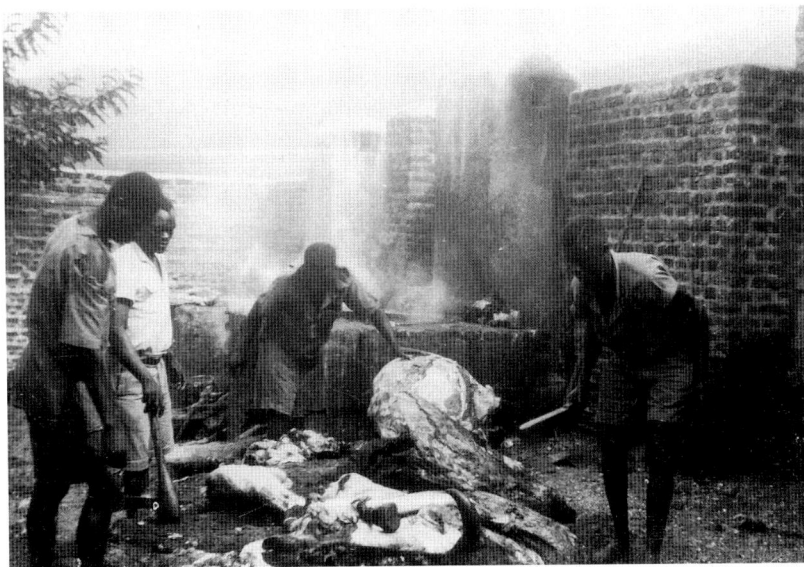

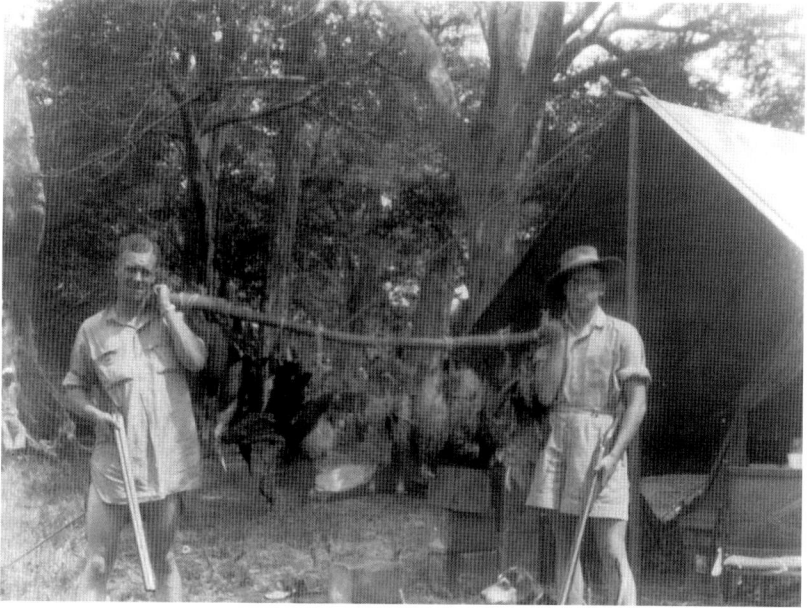

(Above) A bag of Guinea Fowl,

(Below) A typical cattle crush.

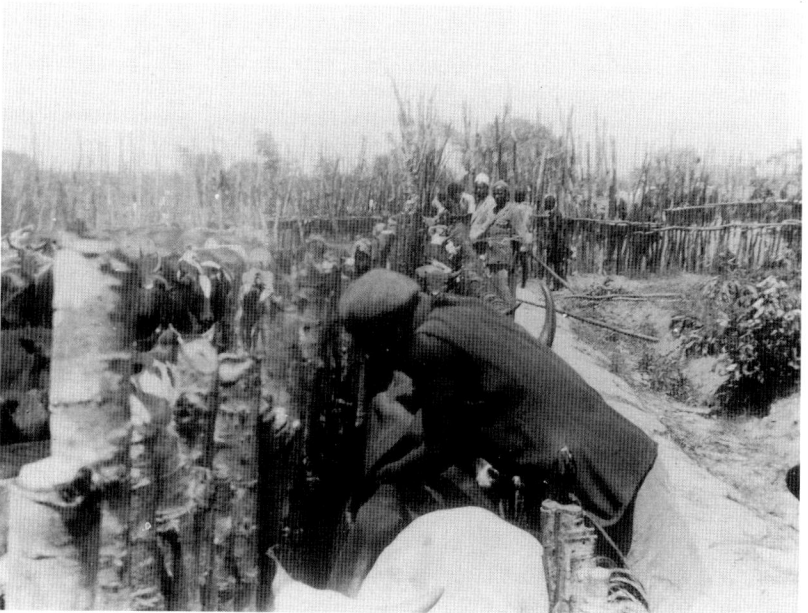

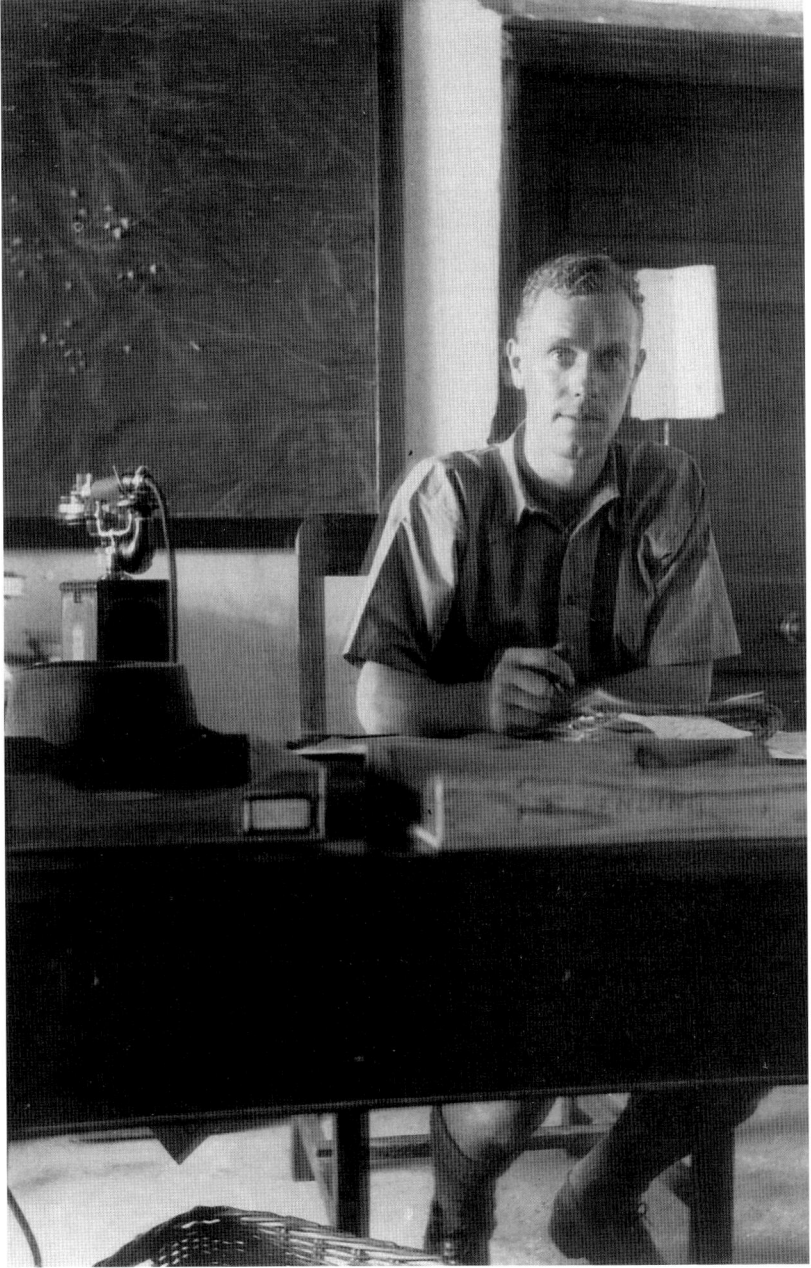

(Above) The author at his desk (filling up the Pending File!), Tabora, 1946.

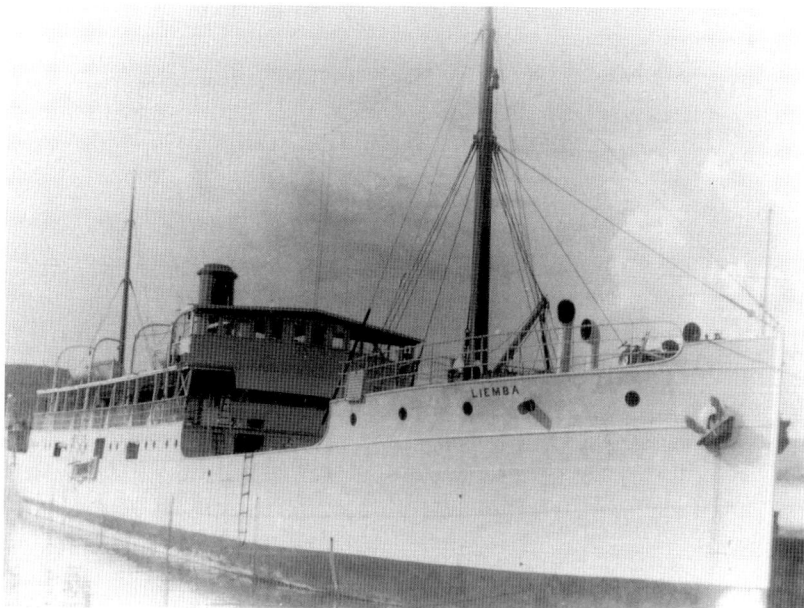

(Above) The S.S.Liemba on Lake Tanganyika at Kigoma

(On Right) Kigoma Veterinary Guard beside Dr Livingstone's monument at Ujiji.

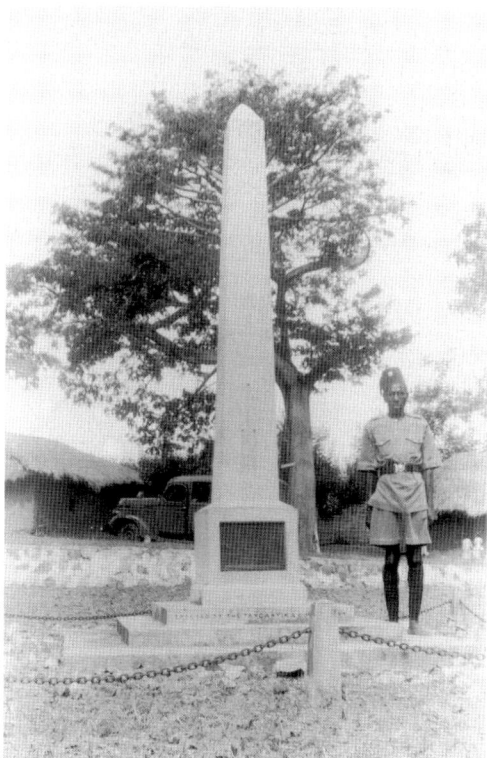

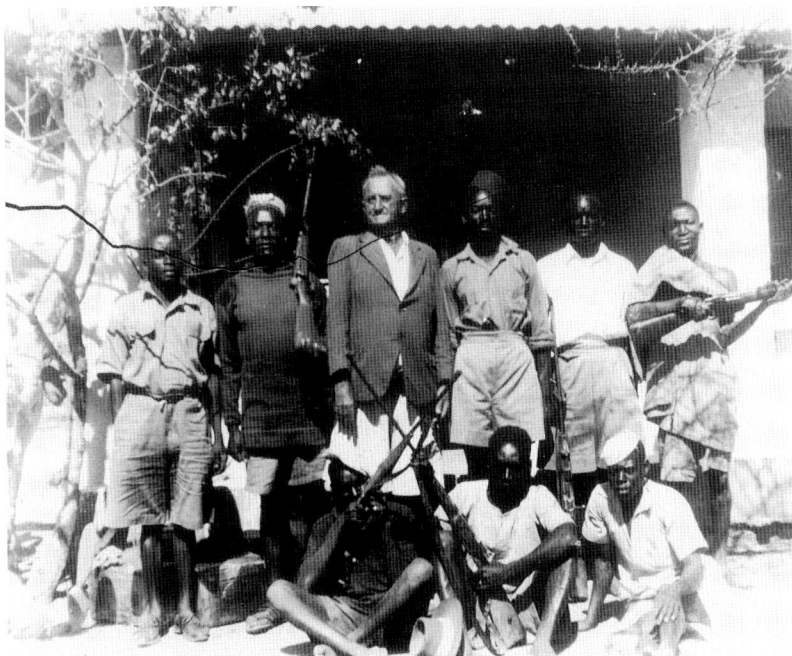

(Above) Mickey Norton with remnants of his private army on the Serengeti at Ikoma.

(Below) Crossing the Malagarasi River at Uvinza, 1946.

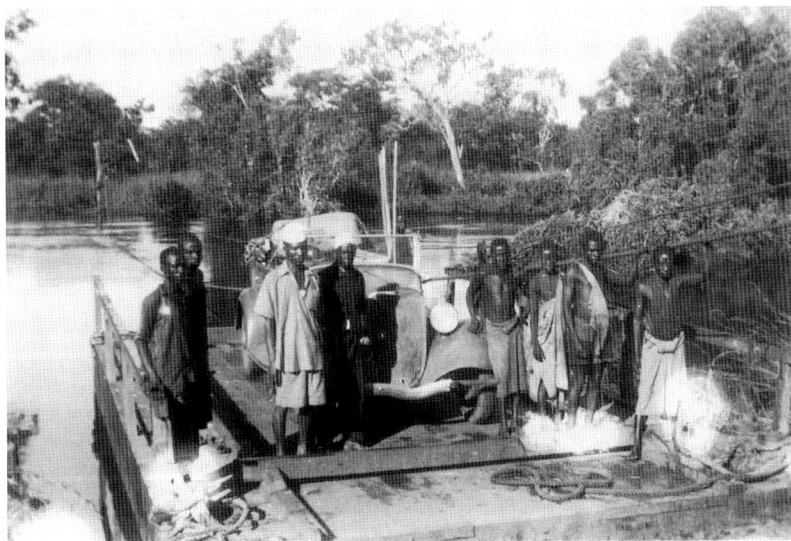

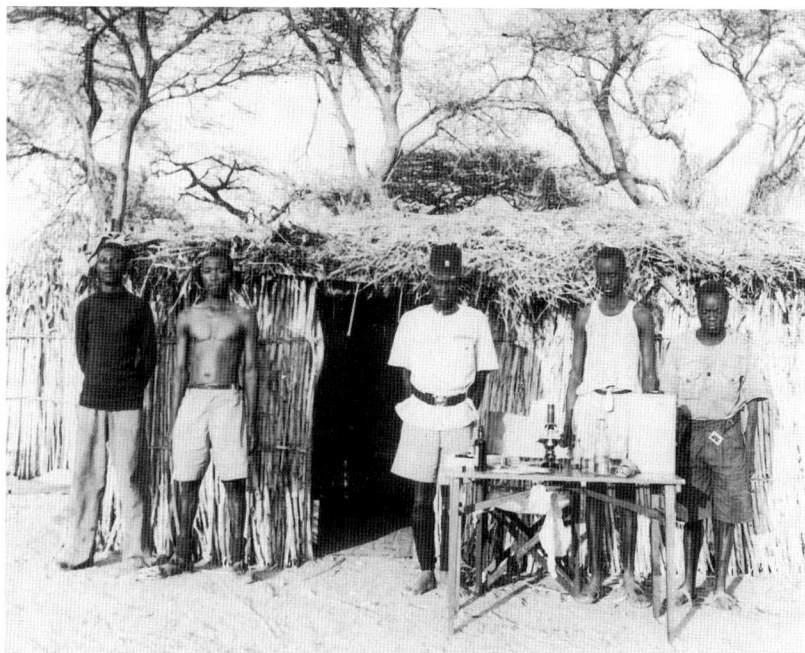
(Above) Field Lab at Bibiti.

(Below) Micky Norton (L) and the author at Benagi, on their last safari together.

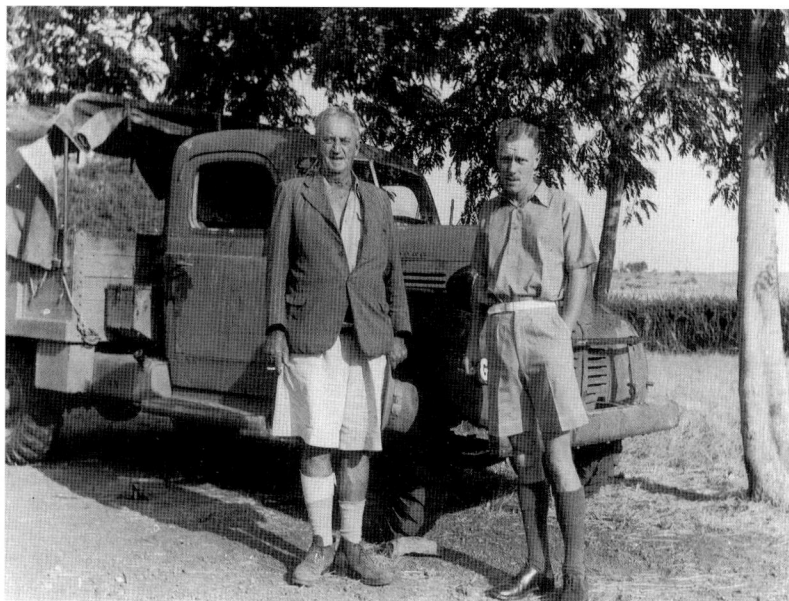

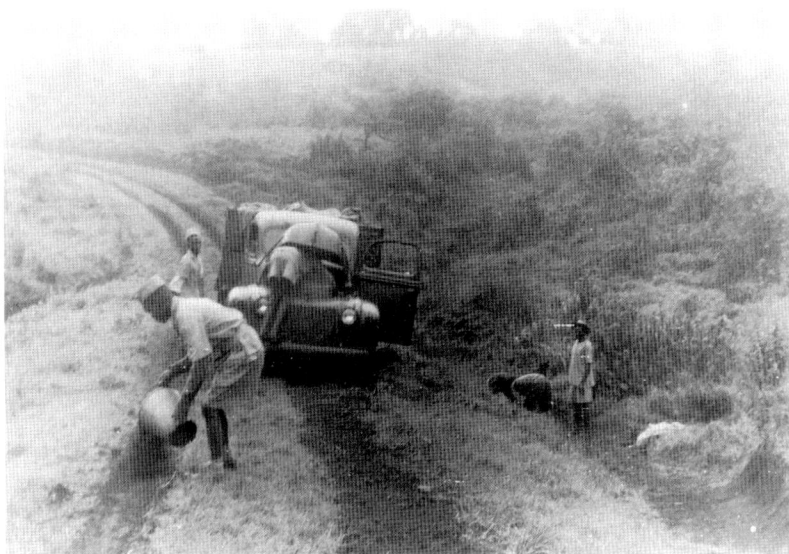

(Above) Stuck on the edge of Ngorogoro Crater, re-laying the road with dry soil.

(Below) the groundnut scheme at Kongwa, 1948.

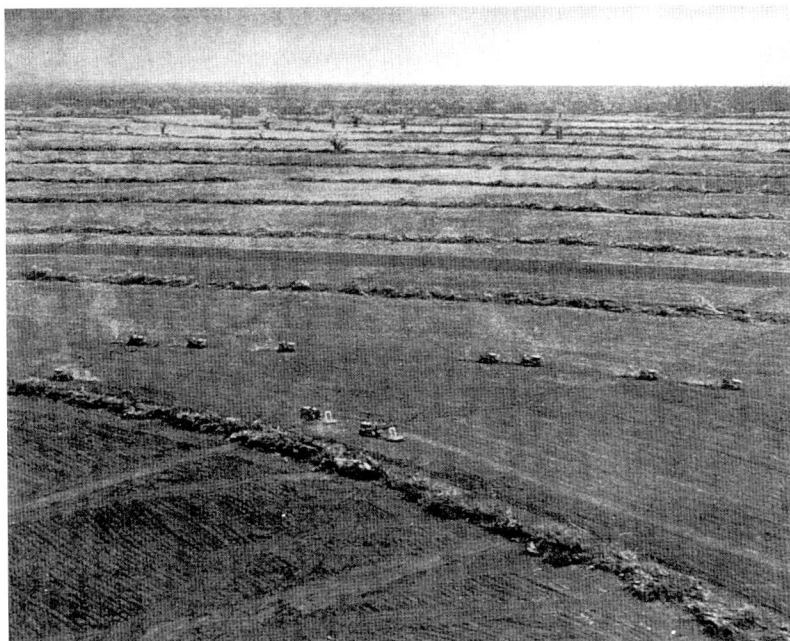

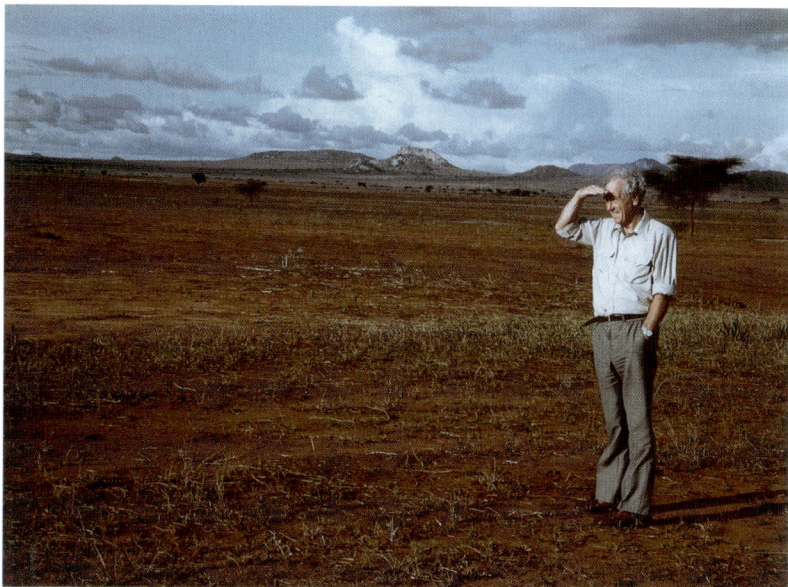

(Above & Below) The site of the Groundnut Scheme at Kongwa, forty five years later, by now devoid of its protective thorn bush cover, grossly overstocked and exposed to wind and water erosion.

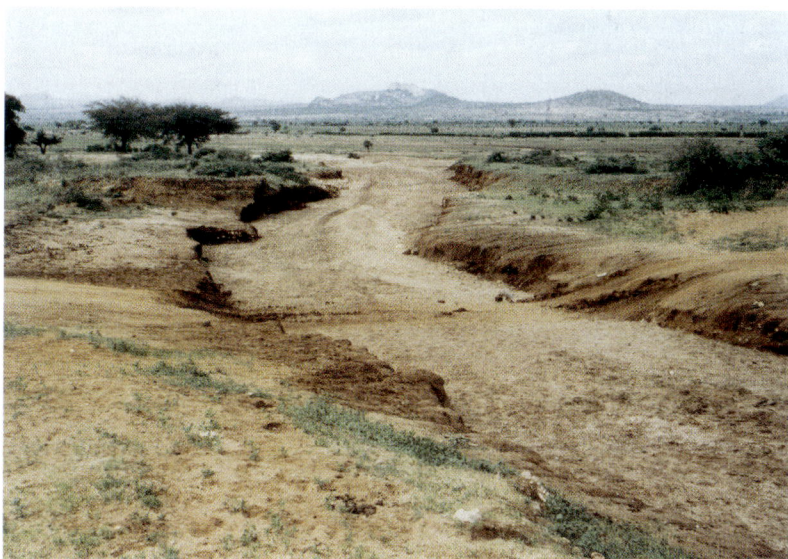

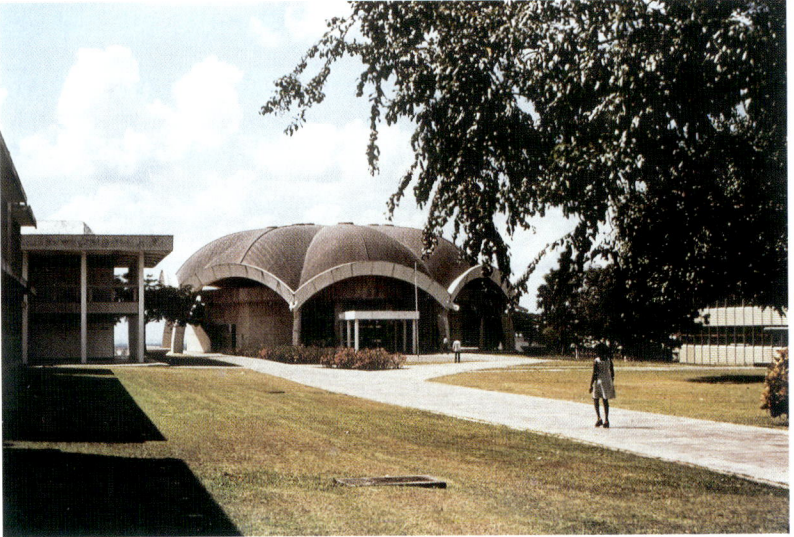

(Above) One of the elegant buildings on the campus of the
University of Dar es Salaam.

(Below) Visiting professors utilising low technology.

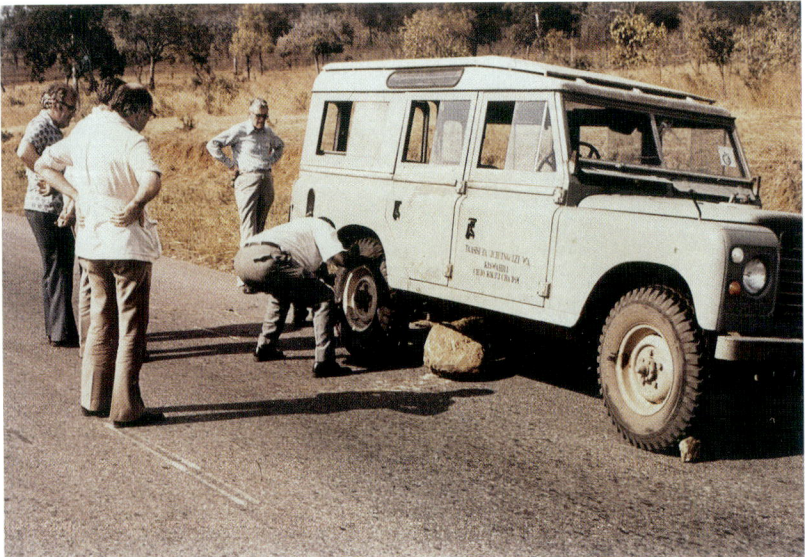

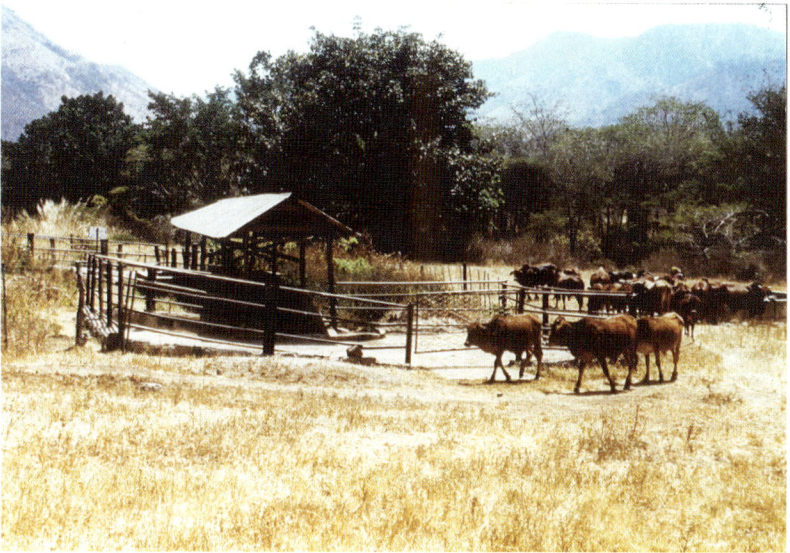

(Above) Cattle dip at Mpwapwa, built 1905 under the German administration, reputed to be the oldest dip in East Africa

(Below) Administration block of the School of Veterinary Medicine at the University of Zambia, Lusaka

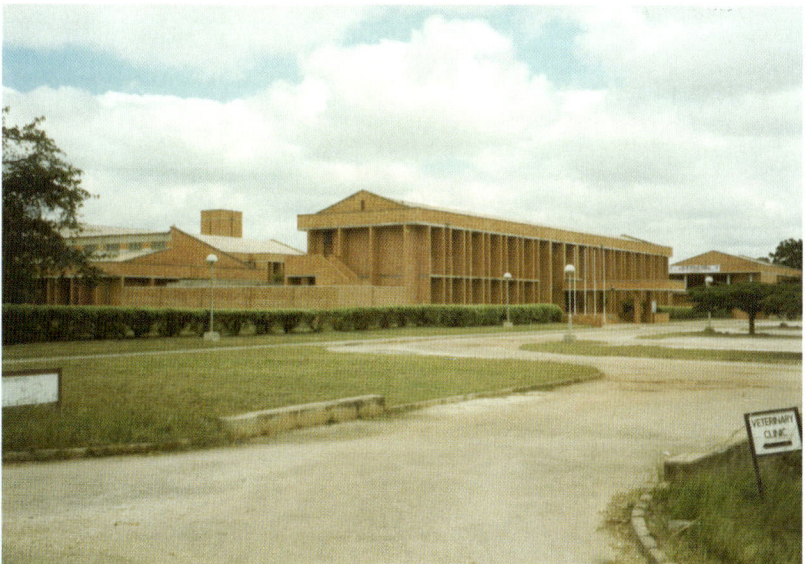

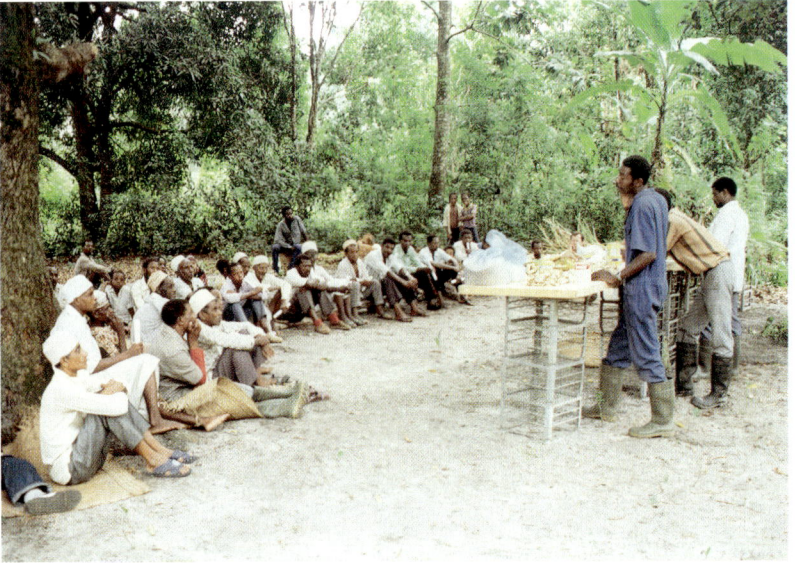

(Above) Extension officers instructing smallholders in practical animal nutrition.

(Below) Jackfruits high in trees, out of reach of grazing animals,
a delicacy for crossbred cows..

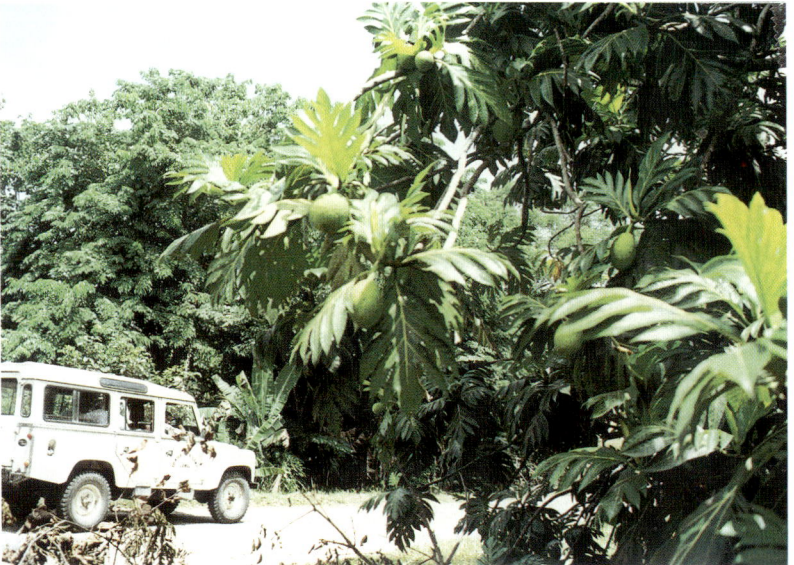

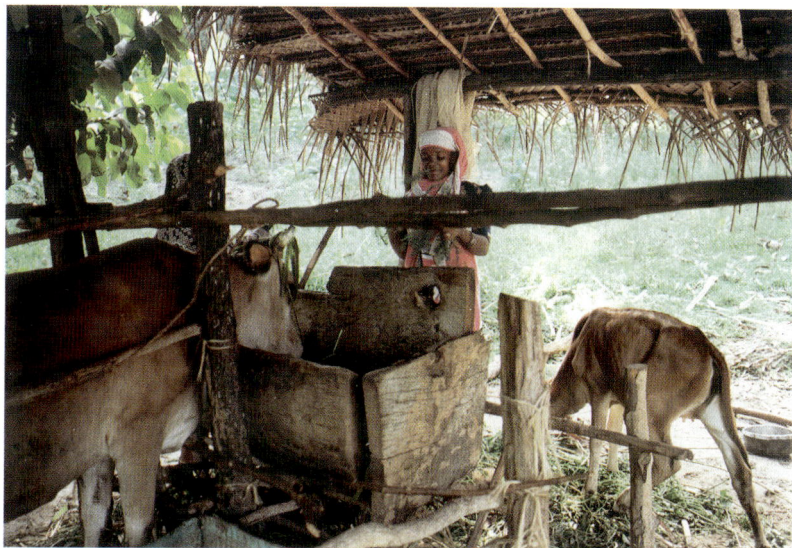

(Above) A crossbred cow enhances the quality of a smallholder's life.

(Below) A resourcefull smallholder.

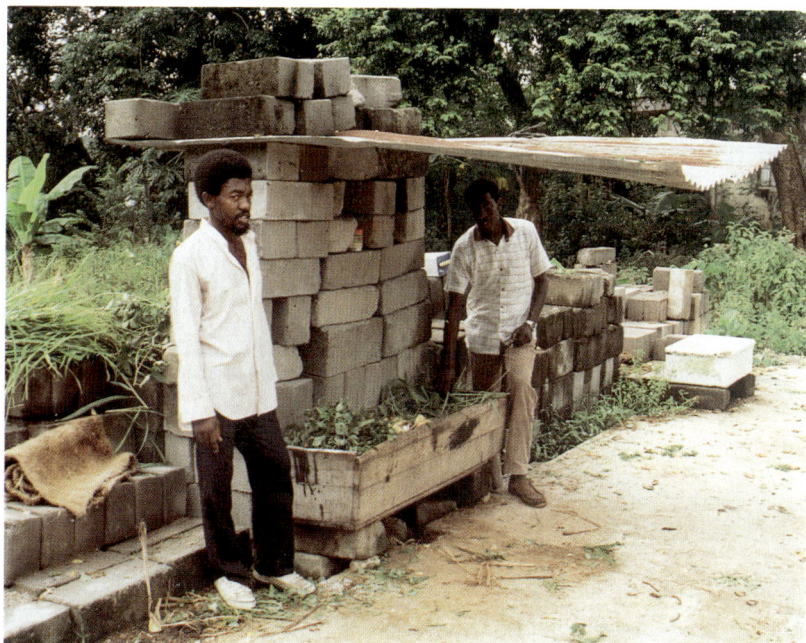

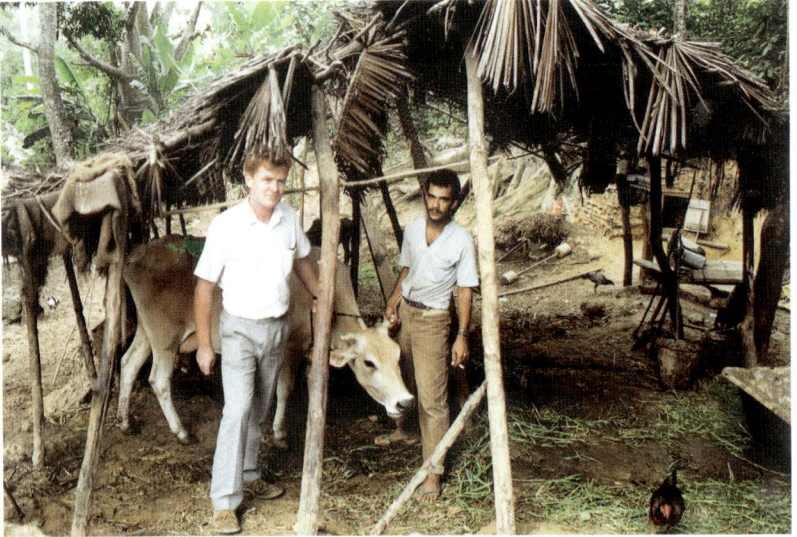

(Above) Outside the Chake Chake vegetable market; the famous cow that peaked at 19 litres per day in her second lactation.

(Below) Son of the famous Chake Chake high yielding cross-bred visiting a village as low-tech substitute for artificial insemination.

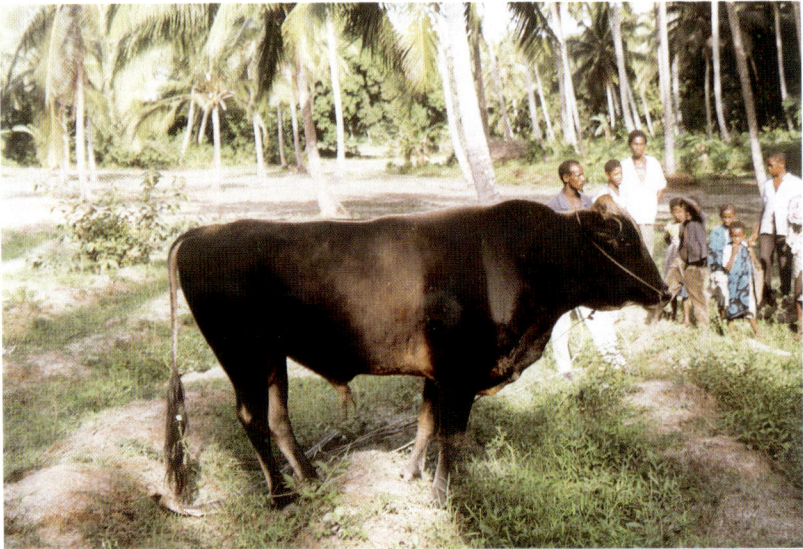

spectacular cases. Several of these photographs were displayed, in the form of 'before' and 'after' masterpieces, in the waiting room which was more like an art gallery than a reception area. For example, there was a particularly grizzly one of an African lady who had been attacked by a leopard that had landed on her shoulders. There were many leopards in the locality and this was a common form of first attack. One arm had been lacerated to such an extent that it was barely hanging on. It was accompanied by another picture of the same lady, taken some months later, happily screwing her head round to admire a very neat stump just below the shoulder. Grizzly though they were, these records of past success may have offered some comfort to other patients waiting their turn. At least the photographs of those days were black and white, several years before the advent of Kodachrome!

The next excitement was a sudden outbreak of foot and mouth disease in our cattle on the Lower Farm that lay out on the plain just beyond Mpwapwa village. In the U.K. and Ireland huge resources were applied to prevent the introduction of this dread disease into the British Isles and when outbreaks did occur the movement of cattle, sheep, pigs and certain other domesticated animals over extensive areas was prohibited; affected farms were quarantined, and all susceptible animals slaughtered. The carcasses were either burnt or buried in quicklime and the premises were thoroughly disinfected. The mortality rate from the disease is not high, seldom more than two per cent, but milk yield is greatly depressed and body condition falls away rapidly. If left uncontrolled, the virus spreads like wildfire so the disease is potentially of great economic importance. In Tanganyika it was not taken so seriously other than on the stock routes, to which we will return in due course, because the milk yield of the local Zebu cattle was only a litre or two a day. Normally, one would have shrugged it off and left it to burn itself out if it had remained confined to the rather worthless cattle on the Lower Farm. To my immense surprise, however, it suddenly appeared in CJ's precious experimental herd in the confines of Kikombo, some three miles away. I was fascinated by this demonstration of the extraordinary infectivity of the foot and mouth virus compared with that of rinderpest, but CJ was not impressed.

CHAPTER FOURTEEN

Time at Mpwapwa
Running Out

Restlessness waiting for the rains and the sudden transformation of the country following their arrival. An elderly French entomologist assigned to the Lab to classify ticks has difficuly in locating the penis of a male! An outbreak of East Coast fever prompts a discussion of the epidemiology and control of the disease. Christmas celebrations and announcement of posting to Tabora as Provincial Veterinary Officer.

Since the hostilities in the Far East had come to an end three months previously the benefits of world peace began to be felt in small ways. I now knew that my brother in the Royal Naval Volunteer Reserve was on the auxiliary aircraft carrier H.M.S. *Fencer* rather than c/o G.P.O. London and that my parents had been able to take holidays with their relatives in Scotland for the first time after a separation of six years. Food rationing was still as severe as ever in the U.K and their letters told of the brisk traffic of visitors from the U.K. crossing the Irish Sea for weekends of feasting on sirloin steak, cream and other delicacies that had never been in short supply in Ireland.

In Mpwapwa, CJ had managed to acquire a mini ex-army Austin station wagon and David White, now P.V.O. Central Province, was hoping to find a car for me in Dar. Cars were still like gold dust so the prospect was inordinately exciting. More and more passages by sea and B.O.A.C. flying boats were becoming available for members of staff who had not had home leave for many years. This aggravated the staff short-age, which was now hyperacute, as there was still only a trickle of new recruits, so it was quite clear that my days at Mpwapwa were numbered. The demand for staff in the field was too acute to allow me to stay on with the Acting Chief Veterinary Research Officer who was expected to return to Mpwapwa after Christmas. There was much speculation as to whether I would be posted to the dreaded humid heat of Dar to relieve David White or to the heavenly cool Southern Highlands where, amongst other delights, there was a chance of meeting a lady administrative assistant or a nursing sister. Old timers such as CJ kept teasing me at sundowners about the loneliness, the huge mosquitoes, blackwater fever and other horrors awaiting me at likely postings.

By now everybody was tired of the dry season and tension was building up; the country was getting bare, there was very little grass left, the cattle were beginning to show their ribs although the cheeky, indomitable little goats still looked sleek. Goats are essentially browsers and a typical end of dry season scene was village goats standing on their hind legs stretching for the highest leaves. The permanent labourers at the laboratory had their own *shambas*, or gardens, so they were getting restive while waiting for the rains to come. Though these were the short rains that lasted just over Christmas into the New Year, they were important because once the soil was softened the *shambas* could be cultivated and planted. If the rains were reasonably good, crops got a head start that could carry them over the short drought to the long rains. Otherwise, the unfortunate farmers would have to watch the seedlings wither away before their eyes and repeat the heavy hand work all over again. They did so with admirable resignation.

The drums in the village had been beating to a late hour, calling for rain, for several days but the labourers had much more faith in CJ than in their own witch doctors. Our met-station was just outside his office and it was he who kept the records. He was continuously pestered for predications and earned his reputation by shrewdly wording them ambiguously so that, irrespective of the outcome, he could always say 'I told you so'. He loved the little game and that year he was over the moon, having hit the target bang on. A group of grateful clients offered him a fine black goat, a colour not easy to come by, but he graciously declined.

One afternoon at the end of November CJ and I were sitting on his open veranda with our arms hanging listlessly over the chairs, watching fork lightning streaking through the leaden sky accompanied almost immediately by cracks of thunder - it was getting very near. The temperature was 92 degrees Fahrenheit. A few plops of rain splattered on the corrugated roof behind us; in no time it belted down in torrents and in a moment we were soaked to the skin. It was so delightful, however, that we just stayed where we were and watched the rivulets of water spilling over the edge of the veranda onto the bare earth and making little channels over what remained of the lawn. After six months of drought the earth in CJ's front garden was still too hard and dry to suck in more than a millimetre or two. The channels ran brown with tiny particles of soil as they grew bigger and bigger. What we were watching was a microcosm of what was taking place simultaneously throughout the length and breath of Tanganyika - soil erosion. Even in the 1940s our Director was greatly concerned and, indeed, sensitive about soil erosion because it was seen at its worst in overstocked cattle areas where over-grazing laid the soil bare by the end of every dry season. Without adequate ground cover there was nothing to hold the soil. Great gullies were cut by the torrential rain and vast quantities of irreplaceable topsoil were swept away. I was soon to learn more about the Department's efforts to control soil erosion after my transfer to the field.

Unlike the spring in temperate climates, the onset of the rains changed the whole environment almost immediately. Next day flying ants were emerging from cracks in the ground just outside my office, spreading their wings and taking off in a steady stream. This attracted a group of labourers and children who scooped them up with glee before they could take off. Flying ants were regarded as a great delicacy. Within a matter of days, the country turned a delicate shade of green; hitherto dry river beds began to trickle again, the smell of wet earth was everywhere and insects, or *dudus,* of all kinds appeared in greater numbers. Spring had come and gone in a trice.

By odd coincidence I was told, just before the rains, that an elderly entomologist would be coming to assist me. This was good news because I never seemed to be able to catch up with an accumulating collection of ticks which kept coming in from the field for identification which was important in connection with the diagnosis and control of tick-borne diseases. Perhaps the new entomologist could also have a go at making our fame with that mysterious barrel of DDT still lying unused in the stores.

My enthusiasm evaporated when a very elderly gentleman eventually arrived at the lab in an ancient box-body station wagon emitting wisps of steam after its uphill climb from Headquarters. He greeted me with *"Bonjour Monsieur"* in a distinctly French accent and as we exchanged the usual pleasantries it became obvious that he was hard of hearing and extremely short-sighted. It subsequently transpired that he had been a collector of zoological specimens for European museums before the war and had recently been recruited by Headquarters without interview as a Game Observer. When he reported for duty it was immediately apparent that despite his qualifications as a zoologist the first requirement for such a post was missing - he could hardly see! The kindly people at Headquarters were in a pickle but he was a charming old gentleman so they passed him on to me as an entomologist.

Next morning I showed him our stock of ticks waiting to be identified and set him up with a stereo microscope, an eyeglass and forceps and suggested that he should have a go at a specimen jar that I knew contained different species including *Rhipicephalus appendiculus*, a three-host tick that transmits East Coast fever. The identification of ticks is a tricky business. There are five morphologically distinct stages in the life of a tick, namely eggs, larvae, nymphs, males and females. In the case of a three-host tick the female, when it is fully engorged with blood drops off the host and lays its eggs on the ground. In due course, a larva emerges from the egg and attaches itself to a passing animal. As soon as it is engorged it drops to the ground and after a while moults to become a nymph which, in its turn, also attaches to a passing host. When engorged the nymph moults and becomes either a male or a female, thereby completing the life cycle. I reminded our entomologist that the larvae, nymphs, males and females each have one or more distinct morphological characteristic that enable them to be distinguished easily one from the other. He seemed to be familiar with this so I suggested that he should start by picking out all the males, transfer them to a separate container and then have a bash at identifying the different species of males he encountered. I left him with the necessary notes containing the appropriate zoological keys and other information necessary for the identification of the common species of veterinary importance.

When I popped in at coffee time there he was with a tick on the end of a tweezers almost touching a watchmaker's magnifying glass screwed into his eye. He seemed rather worried. I called back later and found him even more concerned. "Dees teeks are very difficile, I cannot find dee penis." Oh dear, oh dear; I was disappointed! It is so easy to recognise male ticks - no more difficult than it was differentiating the four young bucks in the practical classes at the Moltino Institue, way back in Cambridge in 1943, from Doris, the beautiful laboratory attendant. She too was morphologically, amongst other things, quite distinct! In the case of ticks there is a hard chitenous shield or scutum extending over the whole of the dorsal aspect of the male whereas in the larva, nymph and female the scutum is confined to a small area immediately behind the head. It just cannot be missed. Trust a Frenchman to insist on finding the penis! Obviously, ticks were not his forte so we eased him gently into a job as supervisor of the zoo. It was also nice to have him around as the father figure of the lab and to hear over coffee of his experiences over many years in Africa.

Ticks happened to be topical at that particular juncture because it coincided with another, more disturbing outbreak of East Coast fever in our rinderpest susceptible cattle at Matamonda. As explained above, the disease is caused by a protozoan parasite (a single-celled organism) called *Theileria parva* which is transmitted to cattle by the bite of the tick *Rhipicephalus appendiculatus*. Even to this day East Coast fever (ECF) is still a serious disease peculiar to East and Central Africa, occurring in extensive areas in Kenya, Uganda, Rwanda, Burundi, Zaire, Tanzania, Zambia and Malawi, which all happen to provide a suitable micro-climate for this particular tick. In such areas it is to this day a major constraint to the development of efficient cattle raising and milk production. The mortality and morbidity rates are high even in the thin, relatively resistant populations of indigenous cattle actually born in locations where infection is endemic. The death rate is much higher in completely susceptible animals introduced from ECF-free areas. The susceptibility of European breeds is such that they are quite unable to survive unless they are completely protected against contact with infected ticks. So far progress has been slow in developing cost-effective drugs for the treatment of clinical cases and such methods of immunisation as have been developed leave much to be desired and are difficult to deploy under field conditions. Consequently, control of the disease still relies heavily on the application of insecticides (or more correctly 'acaracides') by means of spraying or dipping to keep cattle as free as possible of tick infestations. Back in the forties, dipping was used wherever circumstances justified the expenditure of scarce resources to build the necessary dipping tanks.

We had two dipping tanks at Mpwapwa and one at Matamonda. Even with regular dipping in place one shrugged off the loss of the odd animal but this was a more serious outbreak so it had to be investigated. The first step was to look at the dip. A typical cattle dip consists of a narrow swim bath about ten yards long in the form of a concrete tank in the ground, generally with a capacity of 4,000 gallons. There is a large collecting pen at one end from which the cattle are persuaded to take the leap into the tank. The tank is sufficiently deep at this point to ensure that the animal goes right down and is completely submerged before surfacing and swimming to a series of steps that lead from the other end into a large concrete-floored draining pen. Once a herd becomes used to dipping all that is required is for a quiet bullock, with the rest of the mob tight behind him, to be gently prodded into the tank whereupon he is followed by a steady stream of his companions. It is entertaining to watch the action as a mob takes the leap one after another followed by an almighty splash and then to see them surfacing safely and swimming to the steps at the other end. Once up the steps and into the draining pen they invariably give themselves a good shake and are retained there until the dip wash from the whole mob has drained back into the tank. Apart from the need to conserve the wash it was extremely important in those days to do so because it contained no less than 0.125% sodium arsenite – a potentially lethal brew!

Dipping with sodium arsenite at weekly intervals, as was done at Mpwapwa and other centres in those days, could be relied upon, despite the low-tech nature of the exercise, to keep ECF and other tick-borne diseases reasonably well under control, provided the dip was maintained at the correct strength. It was advisable to test at regular intervals and this was easily done by means of a simple titration that could be carried out, if necessary, at the dip site. If the concentration of sodium arsenite was too low the ticks survived the immersion but the cattle died of ECF. If it was too strong the ticks were surely killed, but the cattle were poisoned! Concentration was caused by evaporation so the dipping tank was always roofed, preferably with thatch. Roofing, of course, also reduced the risk of rainwater diluting the dip wash.

In the case of the Matamonda outbreak the test showed that the wash was below strength and it was found that storm water had been flooding into the tank from the draining pen, probably since the beginning of the rains. There was a shallow sump located at the junction between the tank and the draining pen. It was provided with two exit channels, each of which could be opened or closed to divert storm water into a soakaway or to direct dip wash drainings back into the actual dipping tank. The dipping attendants were brainwashed to close the channel leading into the tank immediately after dipping so that storm water would be diverted into the soakaway. This had not been done at Matamonda before the beginning of the rains and when the attendant was taken to task, the answer was the usual '*Nilisahawa tu, Bwana*'! (I just forgot, Bwana). The ticks, classified or otherwise, were getting away with murder this season.

Back at the lab everything began to happen just before Christmas. There was good news from Dar. The great negotiator, David White, had found a 1934 Ford open tourer for me. The price was a giveaway at £100 because a vital part was missing. That was no problem - David knew an Indian who undertook to get the very part. In fact it had happened at an opportune time. A few days later Willie Burns appeared unexpectedly at the lab. He was ill at ease and kept knocking the ash off his cigarette accompanied by a characteristic sniffing of the nose. This signalled that something important was afoot. He blurted out in his Scottish accent: 'It's jist come through! There's a passage for Stutchbury to Australia. He'll be sailing after Christmas. Eh, you are to replace him as Provincial Veterinary Officer Western Province as soon as Wilde arrives.'

I was dumbfounded. I protested that I had spent the whole of my first year on laboratory work, had no experience of the field, had not even been a District V.O. Willie added that I would be all right; there was an experienced Senior Livestock Officer at Tabora who would hold the fort until I got there. He would show me the ropes. I muttered that Western Province was huge, straddling the railway line with mild rinderpest smouldering away; they needed somebody more senior with field experience. His reply ended further discussion: 'That's jist it, Lee! You know more now about the Tabora disease than anyone else. Better start writing your handover notes for Wilde now.' And, kind as ever, he added, 'Don't worry lad, you'll be all right'.

Christmas was on top of us and the pleasure of the run-up to the occasion was enhanced by the arrival of a steady trickle of friends from as far afield as Dar es Salaam and Dodoma who came to enjoy a break in the cool of our mountain retreat. With not a fairy light to be seen it was a much more enjoyable build-up than Christmas carols in supermarkets from November onwards, so characteristic of contemporary consumer society at home. Accommodation at Mpwapwa was no difficulty; our visitors just stayed with friends, where necessary with a shakedown on the veranda. Our way of life was such that there was little formality in such matters and no hassle for either hosts or guests. For example, in the morning guests wandered round in their dressing gowns waiting for their turn to use the limited facilities. Indeed, throughout the year at the appropriate point during dinner parties, in order to reduce pressure on indoor facilities, the men wandered out unobtrusively en bloc to a secluded part of the garden where they stood contentedly in line until the older gentlemen were ready to rejoin the ladies. The ritual was referred to as 'Going out to see Africa'!

Mention of Christmas festivities again brings to mind the fact that life in Mpwapwa did not support the common erroneous conception of the time that prolonged sojourn in the tropics almost invariably led to chronic alcoholism. On the contrary, as explained earlier, sundowners at the end of an afternoon's recreation involved only a pint of lager or a whiskey as did the pre-prandial drink at our dinner parties. But life was busy and, thrown together as we were in the confines of Mpwawa, there were few distractions apart from popping in to each others' houses for a meal perhaps followed by a game of cards, mah-jong, table skittles or darts. When boredom crept in a party would be suggested spontaneously, whereupon the indefatigable Peggy Holloway could always be relied upon to prepare an excellent buffet, our limited stocks of drink would be pooled, and even the more sedate members of the community would let off steam to the delight of all.

One of the most memorable functions turned out to be a party on Christmas Eve which, it was suddenly decided, would be a fancy dress ball. There was a frantic hunt around the houses and the village for the necessary bits and pieces and at the appointed time a colourful, unrecognisable collection of characters consisting of an oriental potentate, a pirate, a parson, a princess, a streetwalker, a tramp, a dock-striker, a bwana dressed as a house boy, a Masai *moran*, a nurse, a ballerina and such like assembled in a vacant house down at the school. The house was brightly lit with tilly lamps and tastefully decorated with banana palms and other vegetation. For some time the music from a gramophone was drowned by the uproarious laughter of the revellers as they discovered the identity of their strange companions. David and Pat White were staying with CJ, next door to me. Pat announced that I was to go as a baby - no discussion. Though I say it myself, she did a wonderful job. At the last minute, I had been dressed in a white laboratory smock tied at the back and stuffed down into a large bath towel tied as a nappy. My long expanse of bare legs were powdered down to my white socks which were tied around the ankles with blue ribbon. A bow made from another bit of the precious blue ribbon decorated my bonnet and the remainder was used to hang a baby's bottle around my neck.

As the party warmed up African drums were produced to support the gramophone. Inevitably, it was proposed and passed *nem. con.* minus one that the baby be christened. The infant was carried struggling to the 'Reverend Pastor' Jack Holloway who performed the ceremony with becoming decorum considering the flamboyant, multinational congregation that vociferously pressed in upon him. The ladies led by the princess, Gwen Reid, then made an abortive attempt to change the baby's nappy. When the party eventually ended six or seven of us squeezed ourselves into the back of CJ's mini station wagon for the journey up the valley to Kikombo. For the baby bachelor Peggy Holloway's nursing in the restricted space as she fed him the last of the Tom Collins from the baby's bottle was a serene end to a memorable party. On the eve of my first year in this strange country so far now from the Christmases of home I was deeply grateful for having been accepted so warmly into my new family of kind friends.

The presence of our visitors over Christmas added to the pleasure of the break but by New Year the last of them had gone and it was back to work with our noses to the grindstone. It was now known for sure that the elusive Jack Wilde would arrive back in Mpwapwa within the next ten days and the Director had decided that I would remain with him for another ten days to ensure that everything was properly handed over. In the meantime I was kept busy writing the Annual Report for the laboratory and preparing my handover notes. In those days these were taken seriously and included a dreary stocktaking of stores, equipment and all categories of livestock which was supposed to tally with what one had received plus an account of all further receipts and disposals. The incoming officer never knew when an auditor from Dar might step off the train.

It was a relief and great pleasure to meet Jack again. I had been very impressed, during my brief acquaintance with him the previous year, by his many accomplishments in all sorts of fields and by his enthusiasm. He was full of beans after his vacation and study tours during the long break at home and impatient to get on with a variety of projects. He was disappointed that I was not to remain with him at Mpwapwa and tried to persuade the Director to have me gazetted Veterinary Research Officer so that my return to Mpwapwa would be guaranteed. His enthusiasm was infectious and I would willingly have returned in due course to sit and learn at his feet. The challenges to which I had been exposed during the past year had brought home to me how much I had to learn. In the meantime I was happy to submit to the insatiable demand of the field for youngsters. During the year my contemporaries, Ian Macadam, Ken Aspinall, Michael Gillet and the two African Apprentice Stock Inspectors, Phillip Princello and Pretorious, had moved on from Mpwapwa. It was high time for me to see the big wide world of Tanganyika.

As I took my leave from the staff at the laboratory one of the most moving moments was my parting from Veterinary Guard Ibrahim who was, among other things, the real manager of the rinderpest *boma*. He was a tall, dignified Somali more than twice my age who had taught me much and, with admirable diplomacy, saved me from many embarrassing situations during the past year. He was a man of few words but as we stood erect looking into each others' eyes exchanging the special three-motioned hand shake there was no need or inclination for either of us to speak. My face reminded him of my great respect and gratitude. His told me that I had come of age and was ready to go. After a touching farewell party I left Mpwawa by train on 22 January, loads and all, accompanied by my faithful Selemani. My father figure *Mpishi* had become progressively more cantankerous and by mutual consent he returned with his wife to the pleasures of the coast. I arrived the next day at Tabora, some 300 miles west, once again following more or less the route Stanley took in his search for Dr Livingstone.

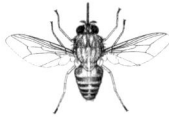

CHAPTER FIFTEEN

Assigned to Western Province

Taking over a Province about three times the size of Ireland; assisted by two Stock Inspectors, three Game Observers (all expatriates) and a large staff of senior and junior Africans throughout the country. Main responsibilities control of transmissible diseases, monitoring game for rinderpest infection, supervision of stock routes and soil conservation.

I was met at Tabora by Mr and Mrs Bailey. He was a Senior Livestock Officer and had been in charge of the Province since the Provincial Veterinary Officer left for Australia three weeks previously after no less than eight years without home leave. They were in their early fifties and I was a little diffident about meeting them because the only reason that I, a complete beginner, was taking over from Bill was that I had a veterinary qualification. I need not have worried because Bill proved to be a big-hearted man who would have readily accepted that wherever possible a veterinarian should be in charge. In any case, he was about to go on leave within a few weeks. By the time we had off-loaded my boxes and taken them to the Veterinary Office it was nearly 10 p.m. When I enquired about a hotel, Mrs Bailey whispered, 'Shush, don't worry, there's a bed waiting for you at Hotel Bailey'. Needless to say, Selemani, according to the custom, was taken over by the Baileys' servants. It appeared we had fallen on our feet. The Baileys were a typically warm-hearted, north of England, childless couple who from the start treated me as one of the family. I stayed with them for a few days and thereafter popped in most afternoons for a cup of tea on my journey out to my own house, generally with a bit of home cooking.

On my first morning Bill Bailey and I went to the Provincial Veterinary Office which was located on a pleasantly shaded road, lined with mango trees. The Provincial Agricultural Office was, appropriately, next door, separated from us by a well-kept garden. Our building housed three offices, a small laboratory, a general store and a garage for the lorry. The staff amounted to three clerks (one Indian and two Africans), a Veterinary Assistant, two Veterinary Guards, a lorry driver and his assistant the turney boy. (See illust.) After introductions Bill took me to a huge map of Western Province on the wall of my office and we reckoned that our territory was on average about 300 miles from north to south by 270 miles from east to west, amounting to 81,000 square miles, practically three times the size of the Republic of Ireland. It was some relief to realise that there were vast empty tracts of forest and bush inhabited only by the tsetse fly and wild animals. Consequently, there was only about a million head of cattle and some three hundred thousand sheep and goats in the whole Province. Nevertheless, it was quite a big practice for one vet! Never mind, there was a European Stock Inspector, Michael Gillet, a friend I had made at Mpwapwa, who was at Nzega seventy-five miles to the north in fairly open country which carried more than half of the cattle population of the Province. There was another Stock Inspector at Sumbawanga down in the south-east, near the end of Lake Tanganyika, and some twenty Veterinary Guards scattered throughout the Province. There were also three elderly European Game Observers who lived almost continuously in bush under canvas. They were assisted by approximately thirty Rinderpest Scouts. The Game Observers' primary job was to monitor the movement of game, mainly in the section of the Province south of the Central Railway line, and to keep their eyes open for any sign of rinderpest infection.

The next item on the programme was a formal call on the Provincial Commissioner, Ralph Varian, who was the senior administrative officer of the Province. Although it was a matter of protocol our meeting was a relaxed affair because he had earlier sent his sick dog to me for treatment at Mpwapwa. Moreover, he was not only an Irishman but, like myself, a Dubliner and we became very good friends despite an age difference.

During the next few days while Bill introduced me to my new duties it became clear that he was a highly organised person. Each member of staff had his allotted duties and the system involving routine chores such as filing, payment of staff, the compiling of information for monthly reports and other returns to Mpwapwa and elsewhere worked like clockwork. This left him free to take me around other Government Departments, shops, the abattoir, and to make several trips into the surrounding country. Tabora, as a Provincial headquarters, was in its own right an important place, but it was also a railway junction with the Central Railway line running straight through to Kigoma on Lake Tanganyika. From there steamers plied across the lake to the Congo and far south to Northern Rhodesia. A branch line from Tabora ran northwards to Mwanza on Lake Victoria and from that point steamers connected across the lake with Bukoba to the west and northwards to ports in Uganda and Kenya. There was also an international airport of sorts, just outside the town, which was on the direct route from South Africa to London. The town itself was a beautiful place, very scattered and placed amongst lovely open parkland dotted with mango trees, a variety of palms, jacaranda and much bougainvillea. Not surprisingly there was a population of about sixty Europeans, which held out the prospect of there being, at least, a few unmarried nursing sisters, stenographers and teachers who in Tanganyika generally were almost as hard to encounter as a gigolo in the convent of a closed order. In addition to the indigenous population of Africans there were settled communities of Asians who mainly ran the commercial life of the town. After the isolation of Mpwapwa it was exciting to visit the Indian *dukas*, or stores, which were gradually filling up with more and more merchandise from overseas. There was also a good sprinkling of Arabs reminding one that Tabora had once been a stronghold for Arab slave traders and an important stopping place on caravan routes for the last two centuries or longer.

I was particularly impressed by the functional simplicity of the town abattoir that was run by the Veterinary Office. It consisted of a large open-sided shed with a corrugated iron roof over a concrete floor, the latter known as a 'slaughter slab', which was raised about twelve inches above the surrounding ground. There was a non-failing supply of water for flushing down the slab which drained into a remote soakaway; in short a spotlessly clean, hygienic facility. All Veterinary Guards were, amongst other things, trained meat inspectors and one from the Tabora

Office attended whenever slaughtering was in progress. One of the most common causes for the rejection of carcasses was the finding of the pea-sized cysts of the parasite *Cysticercus bovis* in the musculature of cattle. If eaten uncooked, these cysts develop in the intestine of man into the tapeworm *Taenia saginata* which is normally some fifteen to twenty foot long, though trophies of thirty-five to fifty foot have been recorded. Though their pathogenic effects are not so disturbing as their length would suggest, the tapeworm can, however, live for many years and the mature segments, each about one to two centimetres long, have a tendency to leave the host spontaneously by wriggling through the anus. Such an occasion can be devastating for the infested person. Picture, for example, the anguish of an elegant young lady in animated conversation with a young man at a cocktail party who suddenly feels a moist segment of tapeworm wriggling down the inside of her thigh. Worse still, such treatments as there were in those days not infrequently failed to detach the tiny head or *scolex*, which is firmly attached to the mucous membrane, high up in the small intestine. In such cases the patient is delighted to be relieved of an immense number of immature and mature segments with the belief that he or she can return with equanimity to the social round. Sadly, in unsuccessfully treated cases the retained *scolex* begins to bud off a new chain of segments and eventually the dreaded feeling of a fresh mature segment wriggling through the anus announces that the wretched tenant is still in possession. Clearly this parasite has to be taken seriously! In more affluent countries, infected carcasses would either be condemned outright for human consumption or frozen and held at temperature below freezing to kill the cysts. In Tanganyika, in the absence of refrigeration, infected carcasses had to be cut up and boiled in disused forty-four-gallon oil drums at the abattoir and sold at half price. Fresh meat was so expensive for the general populace that there was no difficulty in disposing of carcasses treated in this way. Once again, here was an effective low-tech solution to a difficult problem.

The hides and skins were an important exportable by-product. A first grade, shade dried hide was worth about a tenth of the value of the carcass so the Department put much effort into training butchers in the preparation of high quality hides. Similar attention was also given to sheep and goat skins. The traditional method was to hack the hide from the carcass and peg it down to the ground in the full glare of the sun. This resulted in a badly torn, crumpled product which was inclined to putrefy and at best was generally fit only for the manufacture of glue. At Tabora, as at all other slaughter slabs throughout the country, Veterinary Guards provided proper flaying knives and taught the local butchers how to skin the carcass and to remove the subcutaneous fat without lacerating the hide. It was then laced around the edge with sisal rope (available for next to nothing in Tanganyika) and stretched tight in an open, oblong frame made of four reasonably straight bush poles. The frames were stacked upright with a space of about twelve inches between each in an open-sided, thatched drying shed adjacent to the slaughter slab. The circulation of air in the shade enabled the hides to dry out slowly in order to inhibit bacterial activity. When dried and cured in this way they were as flat and as rigid as a sheet of thick cardboard. In this condition they were easily transported to Dar es Salaam or Tanga where they were officially graded by the Veterinary Department before export. Sheep and goat skins were treated in a similar manner.

There were two immunisation camps still operating in the vicinity of Tabora following the outbreak of mild rinderpest, so next day Bill took me out to meet Mr Gibbs, an elderly Game Observer probably in his seventies, who had been brought in from bush to help in the emergency. On the way home I mentioned how surprised I was to find such a gentlemanly old person coping happily with the discomfort of running a camp away out in bush. Bill explained that he was more at home in bush with his small band of Africans than in European company and on the rare occasions when he came in for provisions he could not get out of Tabora quickly enough. He then turned to me and, with a twisted grin, added enigmatically, 'But you haven't met Mickey Norton yet!'

At the end of the month I took over formally from Bill. He had everything in apple-pie order and my only regret was that he was soon going to South Africa for three months leave. Tabora District covered an extensive area but Veterinary Guards were stationed only in localities where there were enough animals to justify their presence. They came into the office at the end of each month for vaccines and other supplies and, although they were literate to a degree, the opportunity was taken to have them report orally on their work. Bill and I sat behind the desk and listened to each Guard's account of diseases such as anthrax, black-quarter, and trypanosomiasis encountered during the month; the number of animals castrated and the state of the grazing. There was a livestock census in progress covering the whole of the District. It was the responsibility of each Veterinary Guard to visit all the villages in his area and record the number of animals in the specified categories. Each month, their notebooks were handed over to one of the clerks who entered the data in the livestock registers. While Bill and I were receiving the census figures from the Tabora District, similar data were being compiled in the Nzega and Sumbawanga Districts and in other parts of the Province where there was any significant number of livestock. It was a remarkably efficient and useful undertaking for a country with such a rudimentary infrastructure. The livestock census had been taken annually almost without fail throughout Tanganyika since the early twenties and was used by Government Departments involved in a variety of matters such as research into the ecology and distribution of tsetse flies, soil erosion, sociology and general administration.

The next group to be interviewed at the end of each month were the cattle dealers - Tanganyikans, Arabs, Greeks, Indians and Somalis - waiting patiently on the veranda. This interview was largely to do with soil conservation, of all things. Recent legislation had designated Provincial and District Veterinary Officers as 'Livestock Controllers'. Its main purpose was to encourage the sale of cattle for slaughter locally, or elsewhere, in areas where the level of over-stocking was such that soil erosion was getting out of hand. The legislation required cattle dealers to obtain monthly permits from the Veterinary Officer/Livestock Controller for the purchase of a stated number of cattle. Permits for the purchase of cattle, sheep and goats in over-stocked areas were issued to many of the dealers, whereas only a few dealers were given permits authorising them to purchase in less heavily stocked localities. The arrival of lots of dealers in congested areas increased the competition; consequently higher prices were offered in an endeavour to tempt more and more reluctant owners to sell. A further control over the system was that dealers moving slaughter cattle along the stock routes within or out of the Province were liable to have their permits checked in order to ascertain the origin of their mobs. By present-day standards the system might appear high-handed on the part of the legislature. However, when one considers the extent to which soil erosion has advanced in Tanganyika since then it is gratifying to record that the Department recognised the seriousness of the problem even in those early days and, at least, exercised itself to slow the process.

Before the end of the month I had moved into my new house which was about a mile or two outside Tabora at the end of a bumpy road right on the top of Kasi Hill. It was a lonely place, there being no other houses on the hill. To add to the feeling of isolation the hill had a reputation for lions so Bill insisted that I take the veterinary lorry home every night. Consequently, there had to be something good on at the Club or elsewhere to induce one to rattle down the rocky lion infested road back to Tabora in a lorry after dark. That is probably why I was offered the house which, with three bedrooms, separate dining room, lounge, ironing room, scullery, store and a multiplicity of verandas, was far too big for a bachelor. It had its compensations, however. Its elevated position gave it an entertaining view, from time to time, of planes landing at and taking off from the airport lying on the plain to the south of the hill. The departure of the B.O.A.C. plane from South Africa on its way to London, the latter only about three days away, tended to exacerbate the loneliness however. On the far horizon, beyond the airport, there was a broad range of mountains diminished by distance to a thin, gently undulating line which reminded one of the immense emptiness of Western Province.

The loneliness was soon dispersed by the arrival of a powerful short wave Pilot radio accompanied by a twelve-volt car battery that David White had managed to find for me in Dar. Everything was dropped until I had the battery charged and an aerial erected. What a moment it was when I tuned in to London and found that the reception was loud and clear! I began to warm to Kasi Hill. Two other luxuries that I had acquired were a fridge and a new cook. One of the office fridges was strictly for the storage of vaccines. The paraffin-operated fridges could go on the blink without warning so it was advisable to keep it at Kasi Hill where it would be under observation seven days a week. This was a blessing because the radio had cost me a month's salary and I was stony broke so could not have spent another month's salary for a fridge even if one could be found. The new cook was a quiet, self-effacing old man who took me greatly by surprise by serving a delicious macaroni and cheese on his first day. My appreciation elicited a wan smile from him as if to say that macaroni and cheese was child's play, and so it transpired. In the days that followed a succession of masterpieces, which included steak and kidney pie, pickled beef, lemon soufflé, crepes, queen of pudding and all sorts of fritters, were served up by a smiling Selemani. From time to time, I caught the occasional glint of the maestro's eyes watching for my reaction from the shadow beyond the dining room door. Selemani had been very upset that Cook Huseni had left him for Dar es Salaam without as much as a, '*Kwa heri ya kuonana*' (goodbye till we meet again). Such behaviour was the height of discourtesy in Swahili culture so one night during an outstandingly good dinner he summed up the change-over by muttering to the effect that 'truly Bwana, that cook Huseni was a right ball-exi' - the latter word, complete with the mandatory Kiswahili vowel suffix!

During my time at Mpwapwa I had lost the most special girlfriend I had known till then. We met at Cambridge and had become wonderful companions but no commitment had been made before we parted because of the uncertainties about the future. Subsequently, a mutual friend had told her that she was only one of many and that there was no prospect of matrimony on my return. Both of these statements were quite erroneous and probably affected both of our lives because soon thereafter she met another and was married. The first few weeks on Kasi Hill had brought the feeling of loss to the surface again but the ministrations of the new cook gradually persuaded me that the indefinite continuation of my bachelor life, even on Kasi Hill, was not quite the end of the world. To begin with I had acquired a miniature dachshund puppy at Mpwapwa. There she was, waiting to bound out to greet me every afternoon on my arrival home. Then I would generally put her though her paces while Selemani poured the welcoming cup of tea. I had taught her a few tricks such as 'beg', 'sit', 'fetch the ball', 'on trust', 'shut the door', and so on. Selemani had been fascinated from the start and had taught her some of the commands in Kiswahili, so here we had a clever little bilingual dachshund, but without a word of German! What remained of the afternoon was put down pleasantly writing letters, pottering in the garden and perhaps reading before it was time for a bath followed by dinner at eight. By the time I sat down with my book, set at precisely the right angle on the table, I was too interested in the delicacies being laid before me and the strains of music from my brand new radio to resume my reading. Yes indeed, there was something to be said for the selfish life of a bachelor on the top of Kasi Hill!

Life did not remain too monastic for long, for having such an accomplished cook, I had no hesitation in asking acquaintances to dinner. Word spread that there were good dinners to be had on the hill and my circle of friends grew. I met one old acquaintance through one of those extraordinary coincidences that bring forth the hackneyed expression, 'What a small world it is'. On one occasion while I was chatting to a caller on the front veranda of the office a rather skinny little soldier shot past on a motor bike and in due course I became aware that he passed up and down almost every morning. Eventually, I happened to get a glimpse of his face as he passed, again heading for the town centre. I could hardly believe what I saw and said to myself, 'No! It cannot be true - I am in Tabora'. But I sat at the roadside for a while and was rewarded by the noise of the bike returning. As I flagged him down I saw that I was right and just said 'Jack Whitworth!' He peered under my Walesey sun helmet and uttered a string of blasphemies followed by '---- Rob Lee. What the ---- are you doing here?' Jack and I had known each other years ago at Sunday school in Dublin. He was the only son and the youngest member of a respectable, God-fearing Dublin family that attended the Presbyterian Church in which I was brought up. His eldest sister taught Sunday school and bashed out on the piano catchy little choruses, which she had picked up from a nearby gospel hall, to the obvious disgust of our ultra-conservative Sunday school Superintendent, a dour Scot who considered any hymn less than a hundred years old a bit dodgy compared with the Psalms of David. We regarded the Whitworths as very religious and would have assumed that his sisters kept Jack strictly on the straight and narrow. Consequently, his introductory string of blasphemy took me by surprise until I learnt more about his subsequent career.

It transpired that Jack had joined the British Army on the outbreak of War as a private and had found his first Sergeant Major less caring than his gentle sisters. Even though he himself had risen to the rank of Sergeant he was utterly disillusioned, a changed man. Clearly his sister's stirring choruses had not stood the test of time. He had hated the Army and here he was, in peacetime Tabora, with absolutely nothing to do! To be taken back to my childhood world by meeting Jack in the depth of Africa and listen almost every day to the noise of my Sunday school pal's bike passing the office was indeed bizarre. He became a frequent caller to Kasi Hill with all sorts of otherwise unobtainable goodies from the Army canteen. In due course, I was invited to dinner at the Sergeants' Mess where he entertained me and his fellow sergeants to hilarious, rather ribald stories relating, *inter alia*, to some of his experiences as a late teen-ager when he played the piano for the Girls Brigade. His more spectacu-lar stories generally began with, 'Luck lads, ya never saw anniething like it . . .' The stories themselves were great but for me the broad Dublin accent made them special!

Ironically, I had heard on the radio that the food situation in the U.K. was as bad as ever. Rationing was still severe and even in East Africa special efforts were being made to increase the exports of tinned beef to Europe. In Tanganyika a scheme with the embarrassingly corny name of 'The Bully Beef for Britain Campaign' was getting underway. The gen-eral idea was to encourage cattle owners by exhortation, as well as price manipulation, in overstocked areas to sell their cattle for the long trek to Liebig's canning factory near Nairobi. The exhortation, as well as manipu-lation, tended to be delegated to Assistant District Officers who were mostly Oxbridge graduates, normally with degrees in classics, history or other branches of the liberal arts. I remember being rather embarrassed for members of the Provincial Administration at a concert at the Club when a young Scottish engineer with a pawkish sense of humour stood up and addressed the audience with his party piece. Being an excellent mimic he launched into a long speech of the kind that was being addressed to villagers at barazas (meetings) throughout the Province as part of the campaign. He delivered his parody at full blast in Kiswahili with an accen-tuated Oxbridge accent interspersed with a little English to run something like this, '*Watu wote, tumefika* hop-ah (for *hapa*) *kuinga mashauri la* low-tay (*lote*) *la* Bully Beef fow Britain Campaign *na mtu huhu*, Bwana Blenkinsop, *ametoka* Economic Contwol Boa-d, Dar es Salaam ...' At appropriate points the Scot raised an arm with clenched fist and shouted a resounding '*assante sana* Bwana!' (thank you very much Bwana) on behalf of the imaginary villagers to express their appreciation. It is only fair to record that the members of the Provincial Administration in the audience that night were loud in their applause!

Another attraction of Kasi Hill was its relative freedom from mosquitoes, compared with Tabora. The latter had a bad reputation for malaria and the whole town had just been sprayed from the air with DDT in preparation for the forthcoming rains. In retrospect, the authorities were extremely naive and happy-go-lucky in the indiscriminate use of this new synthetic chemical that was lethal to practically all species of arthropods, good or bad. No thought was given to the ecological effects of using an insecticide with such a broad spectrum of activity. Furthermore, the possibility of DDT gaining access to the food chain of higher animals was not even thought of. My first encounter with the consequences of DDT entering a food chain did not occur until ten years later in Northern Nigeria. Domestic cats began to die in large numbers in a small town on the bank of the upper reaches of the Niger and the cause was eventually established as DDT poisoning. It transpired that all the houses in the town had been sprayed with DDT during the previous rains as a precaution against malaria. Lizards scuttling across the walls inside the houses, in pursuit of insects landing on the plaster, were an entertaining feature of households in most parts of Africa and they were made welcome by the householders who regarded them almost as pets, though cats thought otherwise. The chemical accumulated in the tissues of the lizards following ingestion of the intoxicated insects. As the concentration of DDT built up in the lizards they probably became lethargic and more easily caught by the cats. In due course, cats began to die as a result of having ingested a lethal dose that the unfortunate lizards had accumulated so efficiently for their predators.

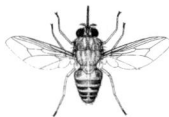

CHAPTER SIXTEEN

Getting Around the Province

Visit to Kigoma at the end of the Central Railway Line and nearby Ujiji where Stanley met Livingstone. On safari again, partly by foot, this time into neigh-bouring Lake Province to check out suspected rinderpest outbreak. Back at Tabora extricating the notorious Irish Game Observer, Micky Norton, and his private army from a contretemps at a mission station deep in bush. Another safari (700 miles in 8 days) in remote country bordering Burundi. Compassionate leave to meet brother on Aircraft Carrier calling at Mombasa.

I was quite pleased to hear from the Veterinary Guard at Kigoma, the rail terminus on Lake Tanganyika, that he needed my help with a cattle dip that had fallen into disrepair. There was no through road but it was an easy journey by train. I caught the up-train from Tabora at 8 p.m. and slept reasonably well in my sleeper despite the fact that one was abruptly wakened during the night by the jabber of people at the few isolated stations. It seemed that everybody within hearing dis-tance of the railway turned out, even during the small hours, to enjoy the excitement of the arrival of a train. The clamour and the happy, shining faces illuminated by the light from the train against the black darkness of the surrounding country was well worth the disturbance of one's sleep. Much of the country beyond Tabora District was practically uninhabited tsetse bush. Shortly after sunrise we crossed the Malagarasi River at Uvinza, a forbidding, low-lying place swathed in early-morning mist. Somewhere nearby there was a salt mine operated by a European and his wife. Though we had not yet met, I felt sorry for them having to earn a living in this desolate place which, amongst other things, was probably rotten with malaria. This was the general area through which Stanley had passed in November 1876 during his second visit to Lake Tanganyika.

In one village he found no less than 186 skulls arranged in two rows stretching the whole length of the village. His subsequent enquiries convinced him that he had been fraternizing with cannibals. Even as seen from the train seventy years later Uvinza was not an inspiring place.

We arrived at Kigoma on time at 11 a.m. to find Veterinary Guard, Idi Abdullah, waiting spick and span in his spotless uniform with buttons and VD buckle burnished bright. I was most impressed. It was a relief, after the dull heavily wooded country through which the train had carried us that morning, to feast one's eyes on the vast expanse of the lake that had opened out before us. It was exciting to realise that away out there, some twenty miles across the lake, was the vast Belgian Congo which stretched across to the shores of the Atlantic more that a thousand miles away. And just below us in the harbour was the SS *Liemba* that plied the four hundred miles along the East Coast of Lake Tanganyika from Burundi in the North to Northern Rhodesia in the South. (See illust.) It was hard to believe that this famous ship had been transported by the Germans in a broken-down condition shortly after the railway line reached Kigoma in 1914. It had been scuttled during the First World War to save it from being taken by the Belgians and was eventually re-floated after the British took over.

But there was no time to linger; Idi had a taxi waiting to take me to the cattle dip and the abattoir that seemed to be the Veterinary Headquarters for the District. On arriving there I found his staff lined up in order of seniority to be presented to me formally. It consisted of two uniformed Rinderpest Scouts, three labourers and a watchman. Despite their orderly appearance the dipping tank, abattoir and hide drying sheds were in a bad state with eroded concrete floors and leaking roofs. All that was needed was a bit of back-up for the Veterinary Guard, who had been unable to get the necessary funds from the Local Authority which was using the dipping and abattoir fees for some other purpose. It surely was in a bad state with the concrete floor of the draining pen badly eroded and a nasty crack in the tank itself. The Indian contractor whom we had picked up on the way impressed me with his efficiency in suggesting what should be done; a price was agreed and after a call on the Local Authority I was free for the day. After a pleasant enough lunch in a fairly broken-down hotel, the obvious thing to do was to drive to Ujiji about ten miles to the south on the lake shore to visit Dr Livingstone's house where, in 1871, Stanley found him and is reputed to have greeted him with the now-famous 'Dr.Livingstone, I presume'.

Even in Livingstone's day Ujiji was a busy trading centre populated by Arabs who lived in substantial flat-roofed houses built of clay with spacious, cool verandas. Arab caravans came to and fro from Zanzibar to Uvinza from which there was easy access by large canoes to more distant centres but, with the coming of the railway and the steamship to Kigoma, Uvinza had been by-passed and had lost much of its former glory. I passed the rest of the day in the company of an old doctor who had sent some leopard skins to me at Mpwapwa for curing. Although the lush, green environment of Kigoma with its abundance of oil palms, mangoes, bananas and pawpaws was scenically attractive the enervating, humid heat on the occasion of my visit was so stifling that it was hard to understand what had induced the old doctor to retire there. Another of those places where a chap would need to be on his guard in case 'a general lack of tone', as described in the Colonial Office's booklet, crept up on him. I was relieved to board the train at 8 p.m. that night en route to the civilisation of Tabora and the cool breeze on Kazi Hill. It had been a neat little safari that had broadened my perspective of the Province, but a more exciting journey which took me right outside the Province had to be undertaken a few days later.

The word rinderpest, especially mild rinderpest, just has to be mentioned at Mpwapwa for telegrams to begin to fly around the country like bees from an up-turned hive. When one, not just a telegram but one marked URGENT, arrived for me I learnt that a suspected outbreak of the disease had been reported at a place called Salawe, in Lake Province, twenty miles on the other side of my northern border. Lake Province had more than two million head of cattle and there was only one Veterinary Officer, Ian Macadam, in the whole area. He was stuck 250 miles away in Musoma District on the Kenya border, dealing with contagious bovine pleuropneumonia, while a Livestock Officer was temporarily in charge of the Provincial Office at Mwanza. I was instructed to proceed immediately to Salawe to investigate. As bad luck would have it, Bill Bailey was now on leave in South Africa and my African Veterinary Assistant, Mr Thabit, had just gone out to an immunisation camp in Tabora District, so I had to get him back immediately to man the office.

The lorry driver picked up Selemani and the new cook, the safari bath containing the cook's utensils, safari box, camp table, chair, camp bed and, of course, my shotgun. As soon as they arrived at the office we loaded a drum of petrol, the tent and some lab equipment and all of us, including a Veterinary Guard and the turney boy (the driver's dog's body), climbed aboard and we were on our way by 12.30 p.m. We made our first stop after seventy-five miles at the District Veterinary Office at Nzega where Michael Gillet was now Stock Inspector. It was good to have him there as I had got to know him and his wife well during my early days at Mpwapwa when he was standing in for CJ while the latter was on leave. He was a steady, well-balanced young man who could be relied upon to deal with any emergency and, as a native of Kenya, he was very much at home in bush. They were a very hospitable couple who genuinely wanted me to stay overnight whenever possible, as much for my company but also as a fourth hand at bridge! There was only one other European on the station, a Nursing Sister who showed a keen interest in me, but only as a potential bridge partner.

Thirty miles further on we came to an abrupt stop at a ford across the Manonga River which is the border between Western and Lake Provinces. Sadly it was in flood so the driver and the turney boy waded across to gauge the depth. It was touch and go but as we had to get to Salawe without delay we decided to chance our arm, as they say in Ireland, rather than trail up river in the hope of finding a safer crossing. The resourceful driver had brought along a bent pipe which he attached to the exhaust. We inched across with barely a ripple, while the rest of us held our breath as the water reached the floor-boards and then, to our delight, drained away without as much as a spit from the engine as we approached the other bank.

We were now in Lake Province heading for Shinyanga, the District Headquarters, twenty-five miles to the north. A few miles on our side of the town we were flagged down by a lad who explained that he was to take us to the Stock Inspector. The latter turned out to be my Africander friend Pretorious, who in company with Phillip the other Apprentice Stock Inspector at Mpwapwa during the previous year, had taken me on many afternoon excursions hunting guineafowl. It was a great reunion. When we came down to earth after a cup of tea we decided that

Pretorious' lorry was better than mine so we transferred the loads and set off for Salawe. From there it was some fifty miles away as the crow flies, but to get here we had to curve north almost to Lake Victoria along a barely perceptible bush track. At 10 p.m., having driven 210 miles from Tabora, we arrived at a little rest hut outside the small village of Mahanga. We decided to call it a day. As we approached the hut a figure emerged who, to our amazement, proved to be another Stock Inspector on safari for some other purpose, quite unaware of the possibility of rinderpest being in the locality. He was hungry for company so after he had fed us we chatted and laughed into the small hours.

My bed had been made up next to a window and soon after we settled down in the cramped quarters a thunderstorm, just as spectacular as they can be at the beginning of the wet season, broke and the rain poured through the window on to my bed. I jumped up and, with the aid of a flash of fork lightning, I managed to close the window tightly. I got back into bed but the rain continued to pour in unabated and when I climbed out once again, amidst grunts and groans from my travelling companions, I found that there was no glass in the wretched window. What a night! It was indeed a one star rest house and even the star must have fallen off!

Next morning we still had a long way to go to the cattle which were somewhere near the tiny village of Salawe. The road had just about petered out so we recruited a local to guide us on our way through attractive, open woodland carpeted with fresh green grass brought forth by the first of the rains. After twenty miles we were surprised to hear a car horn and then spotted a stationary lorry on higher ground a few hundred yards across the parkland to our right. It was the last thing we expected to see in this lonely country. There was a figure standing on the top of the cab furiously waving a stick. As we approached we were rendered almost speechless when we discovered that it was Mac, accompanied by his Stock Inspector, a chuckling Phillip Princello. The reunion in this remote, trackless stretch of bush involving four of us who had all been thrown together a little over a year ago at Mpwapwa was yet another of those chance meetings which seem to exceed the probability of winning the lotto twice-running. Apparently, Mac and Phillip had been down in Mwanza for an appointment with the travelling dentist. Their dental appointments coincided with the fluttering of telegrams from Mpwapwa, so they decided that the opportunity for an unofficial, clandestine dash to Salawe was too good to miss. Wasn't Head Office hundreds of miles away, and Willie Burns need never know!

The stick, which Mac had been waving so desperately, turned out to be the gear lever. It had come adrift in the Driver's hand and the lorry was now stuck in third gear. Pretorious, who was handy at mechanics, managed to strip down the gearbox so that we could send the lorry back to Shinyanga on a slow journey in first gear. Our lorry was unable to accommodate Mac's and Phillip's loads, so all of theirs, except their camp beds and mosquito nets, went back to Shinyanga while the four of us and our combined retinue of camp followers proceeded in our now overcrowded lorry in the general direction of Salawe. Before long we came to a lonely village on the edge of an extensive, flat stretch of black cotton soil. After a downpour of rain, black cotton soil turns into a sticky goo in which vehicles slither from side to side as they dig themselves in and almost invariably come to an inextricable standstill. There was no way we were going to risk being stuck, probably for days, so we parked the lorry and with the help of our guide recruited fifteen porters to take us the remaining fifteen miles to Salawe. The essentials, including a microscope and other lab equipment, a tent, camp beds, camp table, mosquito nets, cooking utensils and, a few provisions were made up into loads, not exceeding fifty pounds each in accordance with Government orders. We were on our way at the head of the caravan - my first foot safari.

Once we were over the cotton soil it was very pleasant striding at a brisk pace through the thinly shaded orchard bush freshened by the previous night's heavy rain. We were soon overtaken by a group of scantily dressed Africans armed with bows and arrows, spears and one or two rather dangerous, inexpensive shot guns called 'dane guns'. They were a happy lot, on their way to a pig hunt. It struck me that, despite the hunters' almost complete freedom from worldly possessions, many an overburdened European businessman would willingly have changed places with them for a few days wild boar hunting in such pleasant surroundings. When the porters began to flag a little the leader of the caravan struck up a song and was joined vociferously in the chorus by the rest of his troop as well as the cheery pig hunters. It was one of those occasions when one felt that if this was work it was almost improper to be paid for it. At about three miles from Salawe we emerged from orchard bush into a wide expanse of flat grassland studded with little groups of cattle that looked like islands in a gently rolling sea of grass. We had made good time and arrived at the Chief's hut at Salawe by 5 p.m. With the energy of youth we went to see the sick cattle while the boys were putting up the tent. The affected animals were young stock and although some were exhibiting excessive lachrymation and blood-tinged diarrhoea all had swollen superficial lymph nodes, so Mac and I felt it was East Coast fever rather than rinderpest. We took lymph and blood slides but by then there was not enough light for the microscope, so we called it a day.

Next morning after a rough night with four beds in the one tent, compensated to some extent by a hearty breakfast of fried bread and eggs - the latter were a godsend and generally available in even remote villages - we stained the slides and examined them under the microscope. To our relief there they were, Koch's blue bodies in the lymph smears, confirming our suspicion that the disease was East Coast fever. This figured all right because the affected animals were all young, not more than about a year old. We were obviously in an East Coast fever area in which the onset of the rains had activated the species of ticks that transmit the disease. Adult animals that manage to survive infections during previous wet seasons acquire an immunity, whereas calves born during the dry season remain susceptible until ticks are activated by the onset of the next rains. Nevertheless, since there was a possibility of rinderpest co-existing with East Coast fever, we asked the Chief to arrange for the neighbouring herds to be brought in for inspection.

The herds began to arrive early next morning while the four of us shaved as best we could with little mirrors stuck up in bushes. Once again, what a beautiful sight it was to see the herds trekking towards us in the crisp early morning across the fresh green plain. With four of us on the job we had soon satisfied ourselves that there was no sign of rinderpest in the assembled herds, which must have amounted to a thousand head in all. We were grateful that it had been yet again a false alarm; we were just sorry that there was at that time no curative treatment for East Coast fever. All we could do was to advise the chief that the herd owners should try to get used engine oil and apply it, by means of a rag tied round the end of a stick, to the ears and the area under the tails of the young stock. These areas were the predilection sites of the offending ticks (*Rhipicephalus appendiculatus*). When properly done the oil clogged the respiratory pores, or spiracles, of the tick and tended to prevent them attaching themselves long enough for the transmission of the protozoan parasite. (In passing, it is interesting to note that the infective stages of the parasite for cattle are not released into the saliva of an infected tick until about three days after the attachment of the tick to the skin of the bovine host.) Apart from this consideration, the application of oil to the predilection sites was probably more effective than we realised at the time because it was subsequently shown that the severity of the disease is to a degree dependent on the quantum of the infective dose, i.e. the number of the protozoan parasites injected by the tick or ticks. Smaller doses probably increase the chances pro rata of the young animal surviving a first infection and thereby developing an acquired immunity.

We were determined to get back to Shinyanga that night so we set off with the porters on the fifteen-mile walk to the lorry. We arrived dead tired but after a drink of boiled milk, kindly supplied by the Chief, and a washing of the feet, reminiscent of biblical times, we were ready for a good meal of mutton and rice. The whole sheep, slaughtered on the spot, cost us only 15c in today's money. Thus refreshed, we drove through the dark to Shinyanga where we arrived at 3 a.m. That morning Mac and Phillip set off on their long journey to Musoma in their own lorry, which had been repaired, whereupon I departed for Tabora after sending my report by telegram to Mpwapwa and Mwanza. Unfortunately, on arrival at the ford across the Manonga we found the river in full flood. When the driver waded across, the water came up to his waist - it was impossible to cross. That necessitated our making a detour of a hundred miles upstream through practically trackless country so we had to overnight at Nzega with the Stock Inspector and his wife, before continuing on to Tabora next day. Such were the exigencies of road travel during the rains.

While I was busy catching up on correspondence and other chores that had accumulated after my six days absence I received the exciting news that my car had arrived from Dar and was waiting for me at the station. I was out the door like a flash and could hardly contain myself when I saw my beautiful, green, open-tourer Ford sitting majestically up on a flat truck above eye level. How exciting! It was not just a very scarce commodity, it was also my first car and I was grateful for the resourcefulness of David White who had managed to secure it for me at long last. The first trip had to be to Kasi Hill to show it to Selemani and *Mpishi*. Its 24 h.p. took it effortlessly up the hill in top gear until we reached the really bumpy bits. The boys were delighted and Selemani just had to climb into the driver's seat to get the feel of the steering wheel and then to screw around to see that the back seat met with his approval. The next job was to put the hood up to ensure that it was in order. That was received with a shaking of the head accompanied by exclamations of, 'Ah, *mzuri sana, mzuri kabisa, Bwana*; oh, oh, oh, *mzuri kwele!*' (Ah, very fine, absolutely fine, Bwana, oh, oh, oh, truly fine). Selemani had suddenly moved up a few steps on the social ladder because his Bwana had a fine car. Back at the office my arrival in the car, despite the fact that it was at least fifteen years old, was met with only slightly less restrained approval.

My euphoria was suddenly dissipated by a distinctly cool phone call from the District Commissioner. He informed me, in a rather accusatory tone, that 'your countryman' Micky Norton (one of my Game Rangers) had arrived at a mission station about eighty miles south of Tabora and was threatening to burn it down if he were not supplied with drink. I was asked, almost told, to get him out of there immediately. Micky Norton was one of the Temporary Game Rangers who had been recruited by the Veterinary Department under the wartime Manpower Order to look for rinderpest in game and to monitor their movements. A few of them had spent most of their lives in bush and were distinctly eccentric gentlemen about whom extraordinary stories were told. For example, while on safari one of them wore a long white gown, called a *kanzu*, as protection against the sun. When a storm broke during the rains he stripped to the skin, rolled the kanzu and his underpants into a tight bundle, stuffed them under the shelter of his voluminous Wallesy sun helmet and strode on through the refreshing downpour. Equally bizarre stories were told about Micky.

I had not had an opportunity to meet him prior to the D.C.'s phone call because he was supposed to be deep in bush away down in the south of the Province. Bill Bailey had filled me in to some extent but during the next six months I learnt a great deal more. Micky had been born some seventy years previously to a respectable family living in Dublin but he turned out to be the wild man of the family and had been sent, probably as a remittance man, to East Africa. Before the outbreak of the Second World War he was well established as an elephant hunter and roved the country with a small private army of Africans armed to the teeth. (See Plate X.) He operated along the Tanganyika/Portuguese East Africa (now Mozambique) border so that he could move from one jurisdiction to the other on the rare occasions when the authorities managed to get on his tail in that remote area. At some time during the war he was caught on the Tanganyika side of the border and was press-ganged under the Manpower Order into the Veterinary Department. At one stage he later confided in me that, when he was caught, he was greatly relieved to know that it was a temporary job because at no time in his life had he ever had any intention of becoming a respectable civil servant despite his family's early ambitions!

My youthful exuberance prompted me to dash down immediately to the beleaguered mission. It was a golden opportunity to go for a decent spin in the new car. This brought a frown to the face of our Indian clerk. He drew me to one side and explained *sotto voce* that this sort of thing had happened before; it could be a delicate business and it had proved more satisfactory in the past to allow Micky's old friend and fellow civil servant, Mr Gibbs, to handle the matter. Accordingly Mr Gibbs was despatched in the veterinary lorry. He arrived back to Kasi Hill the following after-noon with Micky Norton glowering from the passenger's seat and the back of the lorry overflowing with his heavily armed camp followers, sit-ting on tents, safari boxes, bed rolls, four-gallon *debes* (tin petrol cans for carrying water), and other accoutrements. I was grateful that his porters had been discharged, presumably at the mission. Mr Gibbs suggested that Micky and his own boy should stay with me and under no circumstances should either of them be allowed into the town. Fortunately, the Kasi Hill house had two large verandas so the loads were transferred into them, whereupon Micky set up his camp in the less crowded of the two. How grateful I was for the seclusion of Kasi Hill!

When I arrived home the following afternoon I learnt that the bird had flown shortly after I had left for work. Intuition took me to the Railway Hotel and there he was in a corner of the bar almost speechless but he tried hard to articulate that I was a nice young fellow and he wanted to buy me a drink. Somehow, I managed to get him out to the car and home to Kasi Hill. Next morning, I appealed to him as a fellow Irishman to stay where he was and I promised to give him some whiskey when I got home at lunch time. We both kept our promises and that night I gave him another well-watered tot from my precious bottle and continued the treatment for a few days with progressively more water. At least we were communicating and he was soon entertaining me with stories going back to a riotous night on Shaftesbury Avenue when a Chinaman was thrown out a window, thus expediting Micky's passage to East Africa. For my part, I told him about the Dublin he had not seen for almost fifty years and, from time to time, kept warning him about the effects of alcohol on gastric ulcers. In due course, Mr Gibbs declared him fit and safe to be let loose so the camp followers were rounded up, the lorry loaded and Gibbs escorted him back to his designated area of bush. After another incident some six weeks later I entered into a 'Transfer Norton' campaign with Mpwapwa which eventually bore fruit. He was transferred to a neighbouring Province but, little did I know, that was by no means the end of our relationship.

After all that excitement, life as a P.V.O. settled down to the reasonably pleasant routine of office work and short safaris, keeping the inoculation camps supplied with vaccine, moving them when necessary, visiting abattoirs, inspecting work in progress at watering points and grazing reserves on stock routes, visiting cattle markets and laying out new ones, inspecting little bush dairies and so on. The dairies particularly impressed me as they helped the herd owners to regard their cows as a potential source of cash for the purchase of a few consumer goods that could improve the quality of their lives in a small way. This helped them to regard their herds not exclusively as savings accounts for weddings, funerals and other important social occasions. The little dairies were 'low-tech' in today's parlance. Essentially they were milk collection centres consisting of a small house with concrete floor and tin roof. The equipment was nothing more complicated than an Alfa Laval milk separator, a few white enamel basins and buckets, a fireplace on which to simmer the cream and, most important, a supply of clean water. Women from the surrounding villages trekked in every day with gourds full of milk faultlessly balanced on their heads. Their deportment was admirable and a single file of these ladies with heads erect, bearing their loads towards the dairies, gave a dignity to the scene. The separated cream was simmered to convert it into clarified butter which was then poured into four-gallon tin *debes*. After sealing the *debes*, the butter could be kept indefinitely. It was much in demand locally as well as overseas and I was surprised to learn that some finished up in peacetime at Jacob's biscuit factories in Dublin and Liverpool. The little cottage industry was backed up by a rudimentary quality control system headed by a dedicated Livestock Officer, based at the Mpwapwa Laboratory, who spent most of his time touring the country.

But life was by no means all work. It was balanced by a pleasant social round of entertaining and dining with friends, snipe shooting, tennis, hockey matches involving a team of Sikhs who generally beat the Europeans hollow, Saturday night dances at the Club, sipping gin and orange with nursing sisters in the face of huge competition, and occasionally drinking lemonade with a lonely Danish nursing sister at an isolated mission station.

With the return of the Baileys from long leave in South Africa I had more time for safari. My last big one, which subsequently transpired to be near the end of my time at Tabora, was a circular tour of more than 700 miles which took me into a large tract of relatively inaccessible country in the north west of the Province, an area which few Europeans had the opportunity or the inclination to visit. Much of it was tsetse fly country where trypanosomiasis (sleeping sickness) was still active in humans and, of course, in animals as well. It was lonely, sparsely populated country through which a single earth road ran for some 160 miles along the eastern border of what was then Belgian territory, now Burundi. There was no immediate need to visit the area but as it impinged on an international frontier I felt I should, at least, familiarize myself with the locality in case some epizootic disease, such as rinderpest, crossed the border into such cattle as were there or into game animals. There was only one administrative office in the area, which was staffed by a District Officer, and apart from him and his wife and a few missionaries belonging to the Belgian order of White Fathers further north there were no other Europeans in this vast territory. We would be largely on our own so much thought had to be put into deciding what provisions and gear should be taken.

The first leg of the journey was overnight by train from Tabora to Uvinza with the car on a flat truck. The morning mist had risen by the time we unloaded the car at Uvinza. The manager of the salt mine and his wife were at the station to meet, amongst other things, their weekly basket of bacon and vegetables all the way from Bwana Bain beyond Mpwapwa almost 500 miles to the east. It was my first time to meet them. I was struck by the pallor of their faces and, once again, felt sorry for their misfortune in having to earn their living in this dank, uninviting place. Few passengers left the train at Uvinza so their mention of bacon, as well as their loneliness, inevitably led to my having a memorable breakfast with them over which I heard about the country into which I was about to disappear. The country north of Uvinza was named Uha and was populated by rather fierce, xenophobic people called Waha who spoke Kiha rather than Kiswahili. They lived in round huts shaped like inverted pudding bowls which consisted of a framework of thin saplings tied together and thatched with long grass curving smoothly from the top down to the ground. They were reputedly an acrimonious lot and the incidence of murder was believed to be the highest in the whole country. They carried remarkably long-handled spears which were insinuated through the thatch on the side of the hut at the dead of night when seriously aggrieved individuals wanted to settle a score and, like as not, the hut was then set on fire. My new friends advised me not to have too much truck with them in case a misunderstanding arose, especially as their Swahili was not the best.

We crossed the Malagarasi on a pontoon ferry and were soon on our own in Uha. (See Plate X.) The road began to climb and after a few miles we came into more open country and from time to time passed some Waha. They did not look particularly intimidating, though yes, they did have extraordinarily long-handled spears. We were soon in rolling country and the car took hill after hill in its stride, despite the heavy loads, but almost at the top of a particularly steep one it spluttered and came to a standstill. I took off the carburettor and checked it for dirt but found none. We lightened the loads and Selemani and *Mpishi* just managed to push it the few yards over the brow of the hill. With the loads up again we got her moving downhill, jumped aboard, let out the clutch and after a few hiccups the engine burst into life. We sped down to the bottom of the hill and up the next incline, but half way there it spluttered again and died. We were in trouble; I was sure it was the petrol pump and here we were with twenty miles still to go to the District Office at Kasula. I didn't dare tamper with the pump. When Selemani asked '*Taabu gani Bwana?*' (what's the problem), I explained rather patronisingly that on the steep hills the pump seemed to be unable to suck the petrol up to the carburettor – it must have lost its power. He gave me one of his looks and said '*Si kitu*' (no problem) and told me to go up the hill backwards. I was astounded by his perspicacity and my own stupidity! We manoeuvred the car around with the bonnet downhill, pressed the button and after a few spits she burst into life and backed up to the top of the hill without difficulty. For the remaining twenty miles the road wound up and down a series of hills all the way to Kasulu but we soon acquired the technique of dashing up each hill as far as it seemed safe to go, swinging her around as quickly as possible, pushing when necessary, and proceeding to the top in reverse.

We eventually saw a building on the crest of the next hill that proved to be the old German Fort at Kasulu that the present regime had taken over as the District Headquarters. It was a steady, straight climb so when we drove in reverse up to the District Officer, who had spotted our dust trail and watched our approach through binoculars, he was obviously bewildered and impatient for an explanation. The need for the unceremonial entrance in reverse appealed to his sense of humour and got our visit off to a good start. Apart from that, he was delighted to have company for the night as Europeans seldom passed through Kasula. His driver/mechanic was summoned and on stripping down the pump it transpired that the cork gasket was on its last legs. The pump had been sucking air instead of petrol when things got too difficult on the steeper inclines. Needless to say, there were no spares in Kasula so the driver wound lengths of string soaked in petrol round the place where the gasket had been, in order to seal the connection. It did the trick, but for how long? Next morning we set off in trepidation to the next town, Kibondo, eighty miles away, with a few lengths of string for the journey!

The journey to Kibondo was largely uneventful, apart from one intervention with the pump and a rather startling, head-on meeting with a White Father in flowing white robes on a motor bike as we both shot round a curve at a brisk pace. While conversing over a cold drink from my thermos flask we soon found that my French and his English were inadequate so we settled for Swahili. The White Fathers were wonderfully self-reliant, living in remote areas often for long periods on their own. In those days their first tour was five years at the end of which they were given their first and only leave. Consequently, when they said goodbye to their families at the end of that leave they did so for the last time before returning to Africa for the rest of their lives. What a sacrifice they made for their faith and for the scattered people of this lonely country! His was the only vehicle of any kind that we encountered on the eighty-mile run to Kibondo.

As we approached Kibondo we were within ten miles of the Burundi border and enjoyed the views of the rolling grassland hills characteristic of those parts. To the east of our road were miles upon miles of heavily wooded tsetse bush. Kibondo was much more of a town than Kasulu with a few Indian *dukas* and a goodly population of Africans. Much excitement was created by the arrival of our car, especially as it was driven by a *Mzungu* (European), and we were accompanied into the town by a cheery crowd of children doing their best to keep abreast of us at either side of the car. When we stopped in a wide open space in the centre everyone within sight converged on us and stood in a circle around the car. Greetings were exchanged and when I got out one gentleman came forward, drew himself smartly to attention, saluted with a stamp of his right foot and said, '*Jambo Bwana Mganga*' (greetings doctor). To my surprise I saw the VD on his belt and realised that this was the Veterinary Guard whom I had come to visit. When a suitable opportunity arose I asked why he was not in uniform, he explained that his puttees, tunic and fez had long since worn out and he had received no response to his many requests to Tabora for replacements. I then expressed my surprise as to why he had not told the last person who had come through from Tabora. He explained that his uniform was fine then. 'How long ago was that?' I enquired. 'Seven years, Bwana'!

Despite the neglect he seemed to be attending to his duties well, entirely on his own initiative. Kibondo was a so-called sleeping sickness settlement. It was surrounded by tsetse fly bush in which the trypanosomes responsible for sleeping sickness in humans and *negana* in animals were prevalent. Extensive area around the town had been cleared to deprive the tsetse flies of the shade which was essential for their survival. Unfortunately, herdsmen and their animals grazing near the periphery of the cleared land were liable to become infected, as were those who went into bush for firewood; honey hunters put themselves at even greater risk. There was a little clinic staffed by a Medical Orderly who, in addition to looking after the general health of the human population, was responsible for the diagnosis and treatment of sleeping sickness. When I visited the clinic I found that the Veterinary Guard and his medical confrere were great pals and virtually shared the clinic. They shared the same microscope and hypodermic syringes and both of them rose in my admiration when they showed me the latter. These were the ubiquitous Record syringes, now obsolete, which consisted of a glass barrel with a nickel disc at one end which carried the needle. The top of the barrel fitted into another nickel disc with a hole in the centre which guided the metal rod of the plunger. To my amazement the glass barrels of all the 'useable' syringes were shattered at the top, presenting sharp spikes; that is, the whole thing was devoid of the top disk which served to keep the plunger steady and in line. The Orderly and the Veterinary Guard were reduced to having to use them for, mark you, intravenous injections in both man and animals and they complained that it was very difficult to get them into the veins and keep them steady without lacerating themselves, especially when dealing with a nervous child or a bucking bullock! I marvelled at their stoicism; they were an admirable pair and I resolved to do my utmost to see that they were cared for in the manner they deserved.

When I expressed my concern about setting off on the next leg of my journey with a faulty petrol pump the Veterinary Guard took me to the house of a trader, one of the few Indians in the town, who ran a couple of Ford lorries. After a courteous welcome I explained my problem and was taken into the adjoining shop. There, hanging on a nail in the wall was a cork gasket. To this day I can see it, the only one on the whitewashed wall and it was exactly the size I needed for the petrol pump. To me it was like gold dust and, to my embarrassment, the kind trader insisted that I take it with his compliments. Thereafter, the journey to the District Veterinary Office at Singida through the town of Kahama was largely uneventful. It was just a question of slogging along the 250 miles of bumpy road and, from time to time, pushing where it had been washed away since the rains began. It was an easy seventy-five miles from there to Tabora, making in all a round trip of some 700 miles by train and road in eight days. No wonder the Veterinary Guard had had to wait seven years for a new uniform!

Ironically, shortly after my return to Tabora, feeling that I now had a reasonable knowledge of the northern half of the Province and looking forward to a trip on the *Liemba* to the southern end of Lake Tanganyika, I heard that I was soon to be transferred elsewhere. My old friend Sandy Milne, who had introduced me to this new life when I disembarked from the *Straat Soenda* at Dar es Salaam eighteen months previously, was due back from home leave and was to take over the Province within a few weeks. Before I had time to consider whether that suited me or not a much more exciting telegram arrived from my brother telling me that the aircraft carrier, H.M.S. *Fencer*, on which he was the Surgeon Lieutenant, would be putting into Mombasa on 11 June, the following week, on its homeward voyage from Ceylon. There was no time to lose; with tongue in cheek I shot off a telegram to Mpwapwa. With characteristic no-messing kindness one arrived back by return from Headquarters telling me to hand over to Bill Bailey, as soon as I wished, and take fourteen days leave - more if necessary. I was a bit vague as to how to get to Mombasa but as it was on the coast I jumped on the next down-train and was in Dar es Salaam the following day. My first call was to David White and his wife Pat. Their house was in a shambles as they were packing up, having been given seats at short notice on the British Overseas Airways Flying Boat which did the reputedly delightful journey to England in a leisurely five days. When I saw them off next morning the resourceful David, whom everybody regarded as the Department's fixer, had got a seat for me on a small plane flying to Mombasa two days later. Dar es Salaam was at its best in June, with the rains and clammy humidity behind it. It was wonderful after eighteen months to feel the bustle of Dar and to see the wide expanses of the Indian Ocean which, amongst other things, gave one a feeling of contact with the outside world after the remoteness of Western Province. To this was added the relief of having no responsibilities and no decisions more difficult to make than whether to swim at Oyster Beach, or just sit over a cold beer on the veranda of the original New Africa

Hotel. From the veranda one could watch the busy world of rickshaws, heavily laden hand carts pushed by Swahilis stripped to the waist, Arabs in white *kanzus*, sun-helmeted Europeans and turbaned Sikhs, passing by.

The 'airport' to which I and my fellow passengers were driven two days later was little more than a flying field with a few sheds. I had never flown before and so was quite excited at the prospect. The plane was a smart seven-seater biplane. We taxied down the field, then raced into the wind and almost immediately we were soaring high over Dar es Salaam, fascinated by the different shades of green of the coconut plantations, sisal estates, and lawns; the brown stubble of cultivated patches; the red roofs; and then, the brilliant silver of the beach at Oyster Bay; followed by the calm, azure sea, its colour broken with patches of light green and yellow over submerged coral reefs. The flight to Mombasa via Zanzibar and Tanga took us just over two hours, including stopping time, compared with at least two days by road. It was a foretaste of how air travel was soon going to speed up travel within Tanganyika even more spectacularly than the railways had done less than forty years previously.

Mombasa was a world different from anything I had experienced since Durban - five course meals in the Manor Hotel, wash-hand basins in the bedroom, tarmacadam roads, buses, real shops and daily newspapers. I heard that the S.S. *Madura,* en route from England to Dar es Salaam, was in the harbour so I went down to have a look at the passenger list and was delighted to find that Sandy Milne, who was to take over from me within a few weeks, was on board. So too was Colin Browne, another Veterinary Officer returning to Tanganyika after home leave in Ireland. Colin had been a few years ahead of me at the Veterinary College. Our meeting gave me the run of the ship and we had a wonderful weekend exchanging news, playing deck tennis, swimming and overall enjoying Sandy's hilarious sense of humour. The *Madura* left just before the *Fencer*'s arrival on Tuesday. The *Fencer* was an impressive sight as she entered the harbour and while the gap between her and the wharf narrowed, I peered along the rows of crew and passengers lining the rails in the hope of spotting my brother. Suddenly, I spotted Angus and discovered that the crafty fellow had been watching my activities for some time with camera at the ready. I am afraid my delight was rather more unrestrained than his; fittingly so, after all he was my big brother and was under the watchful eye of his fellow officers and able-bodied seamen. He smiled benevolently as he introduced me to the Captain and his fellow officers; then, as soon as we were in the privacy of his cabin, beaming from cheek to cheek, he put his arm around my shoulder and, said, 'Gee Boy, this is fantastic, how the divil are you?' The 'Gee' was a schoolboy corruption of our surname given to both of us by our respective classmates. He was indeed an elder brother, one who had been getting me out of scrapes and leading me into others since childhood.

Back in the Ward Room over pink gins, the Commander kindly invited me to spend the next three nights on board. The Ward Room, like the rest of the ship, was looking tired and tatty after its war service. She was one of the first small aircraft carriers that had been mass-produced in the United States and handed over to the Royal Navy under the Lease Lend Scheme just before Pearl Harbour. She had been engaged mainly as an escort ship for convoys and at the end of hostilities in the Far East she was converted into a troop-carrier with serried ranks of bunks, four or five storeys high, in the hangers below deck. Two shifts of passengers occupied the bunks every twenty-four hours, those using the upper levels having to climb up ladders provided for the purpose and presumably strapping themselves in. Thus equipped, the *Fencer* was being used for the repatriation of servicemen and women from the Far East to England, prior to their demobilisation. On each homeward voyage she carried hundreds of passengers. It was a tough journey in the tropical heat in such congested conditions and there was a good deal of illness resulting from the recurrence of malaria and other tropical diseases. The passengers were tired and just wanted to get home. It seemed a heavy responsibility for a relatively inexperienced Surgeon Lieutenant to be responsible for the health of so many under these conditions but that was par for the course during the aftermath of the war. There were a few elderly people in the sickbay who, though seriously ill, insisted on continuing their journey rather than being transferred ashore. I noticed how he kept them uppermost in his mind, spending a goodly time with them before going ashore and seeing them again as soon as he returned. He explained his philosophy, one that he held dear to the end of his busy career: the outcome of a serious illness so often depended on the sheer energy that one was prepared to put into the case.

After three wonderful days living almost as one of the crew it was time for me to catch the plane and as I flew across the harbour I got my last view of the aircraft carrier, now like a child's toy on a pond far beneath me. It was hard to believe that life still went on below its decks and that my brother was actually in the middle of it all, heading home. Next day, on boarding the train for the two-day journey from Dar es Salaam to Tabora I was delighted to find that Sandy Milne and Colin Browne were my travelling companions. Colin was in great form, being on his way to take over Southern Highlands Province, a much-prized posting because of its cool climate and the beauty of the countryside. For my part, it was good to know that I could now pass the buck to Sandy if things got too hot before my departure from Tabora.

Indeed, a few days later I completely handed over the Province to Sandy. The instructions from Mpwapwa were that I was to travel by train with my car and loads to Mwanza, the Provincial Headquarters of Lake Province, where Carl Anderson, a Senior Livestock Officer, was to remain in administrative charge until the return of Stutchbury from home leave in Australia. He was to take over then. In the intervening time I was to travel throughout the various Districts of Sukumaland so that I would be familiar with the country in preparation for the investigation of any outbreaks of disease that might occur. It seemed an interesting assignment. The livestock population of Lake Province was the highest in the country, the Province having more than two million head of cattle, a million sheep and over a million goats, the vast majority of which were in Sukumaland. By and large Sukumaland was relatively treeless, bare, rolling grassland which supported cotton growing as well as livestock. With such a large livestock population it was obviously sensible to have two Veterinary Officers: Mac in Musoma District to the north on the Kenya border (where he was tied down with a large pleuropneumonia immunisation campaign); and me, largely free of administrative duties in Sukumaland in the centre of the Province. I set about saying my goodbyes and prepared leisurely for my departure at the end of June but within a few days telegrams began to fly again. There was a suspected outbreak of rinderpest at Hendawashi, a tiny, isolated village on the Sibiti plains near Lake Eyasi in the remote south-eastern corner of Lake Province. The locality was so little known that precise map references were quoted in the telegrams. I was to get across the border to Shinyanga immediately where I was to pick up a suitable truck, as well as Micky Norton, whose services were to be at my disposal. Dear, oh dear! My 'Transfer Micky Norton Campaign' had backfired!

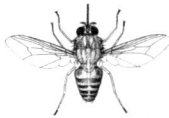

CHAPTER SEVENTEEN

Bushwhacking Through Lake Province

On continuous safari for three months throughout the Province in search of rinderpest. Inspected up to 40,000 head of cattle along the Sibiti River, witnessing the appalling effects of drought on the people, their cattle, and the integrity of the soil on the vast Sibiti Plains. Encountered and dealt with foot and mouth disease on the stock routes leading eventually to Nairobi. Around Lake Victoria to Bukoba still on the rinderpest trail to investigate cattle floatng down a river from Rwanda (the same river that would have human bodies floating down it 52 years later). Preparing for a safari across the Serengetti.

On arrival at Shinyanga the following day, where my young friend Pretorius was still in charge of the District Veterinary Office, I learnt that the reported outbreak had been a false alarm. It had been reported to Mpwapwa by telegram and already there was an angry reply from Civet (the telegraphic address of the Director of Veterinary Services) addressed to Provet, the Provincial Veterinary Office at Mwanza, copied to 'Uncle Tom Cobley and All', demanding to know who had reported the outbreak, who had sent the telegram addressed to Shinyanga instead of Maswa, where was Micky Norton, and much else besides. This prickliness was probably aggravated by the drought of 1946, which was affecting man as well as animals progressively as the year wore on.

As early as February, following a failure of the short rains at the end of 1945, the Provincial Administration, assisted by staff members of the Agricultural and Veterinary Departments in Western Province and, no doubt, elsewhere, had been taking every opportunity to urge chiefs and village leaders to encourage their people to plant greater reserves of drought-resistant crops, such as cassava and millet, in case the main rains proved insufficient for maize, the preferred crop. As it subsequently transpired the long rains, which normally begin at the end of February/early March were scanty and badly distributed. This, incidentally, had added a further stimulus for de-stocking which was an integral part of the so-called Bully Beef Campaign. By the time I reached Shinyanga at the end of June, the drought was beginning to bite and I was about to see the disastrous consequences this was having for the cattle populations of Lake Province north of the Manonga and Sibiti Rivers and as far to the east as Lake Eyasi. Grass was becoming progressively scarcer on parts of the Serengeti Plains and to complicate matters further, there were several foci of rinderpest in game in Northern Province and some of these herds were moving southwards towards Lake Eyasi and Central Province. Little wonder Mpwapwa was testy about false alarms at Hendawashi; the cattle populations in that general area were obviously seriously at risk. Accordingly, I was now instructed to inspect cattle along the whole country to the north of the Manonga and Sibili Rivers through to Lake Eyasi. It was going to be a tough safari, so a rugged ex-army desert truck was sent down to me from Mwanza. By then I had arranged for Micky Norton to patrol areas of tsetse bush, to the north-east of my route, into which game were possibly moving from Northern Province.

I set off at the beginning of July with Selemani, *Mpishi*, a Veterinary Guard, two Rinderpest Scouts and, of course, a driver and his turney boy. As we would be out of touch with the outside world for two or three weeks it was necessary to take along a spare 44-gallon drum of petrol, camp equipment and provisions for the eight of us - a considerable load. The journey to Lake Eyasi would be about one hundred miles as the crow flies. We would then swing up to a camp on the stock routes at Kimali some forty miles north near the south-eastern edge of the Serengeti Plains. From there we would drive sixty miles westwards to the tiny town of Shanwa. Shanwa was the headquarters of Maswa District and as such it had a small European community. This consisted of three bachelors, namely an Assistant District Officer, a Works Foreman and a young, inexperienced Stock Inspector recently arrived from England. Though it was away out in bush seventy-five miles from Mwanza, letters and telegrams could be sent from there so that was to be my next point of contact for communicating with Mwanza and Mpwapwa.

We made fifty miles the first day to Karitu on the Manonga River and pitched the tents at a delightful, shaded site overlooking a stretch of the river where there was a variety of water fowl to entertain us, as well as pelicans in a nearby tree. Almost immediately, the *Jumbe* or headman from the nearby village, accompanied by some of the elders and the usual entourage of curious women and children, arrived to greet us. After the formal handshakes and arrangements for water, firewood and the purchase of a sheep for the pot had been made, the Veterinary Guard and I asked about the health of the animals in the surrounding country. There seemed to be no major problem other than drought so we then discussed our plan of campaign for the next few days, namely that the herds should be brought in to a central point near the camp from the villages or *boma*s within half a day's walk. Simultaneously, the Rinderpest Scouts would visit the respective *boma*s to ascertain that no calves or sick cows had been left behind and to look for unusual numbers of hides or perhaps skeletons. These arrangements were welcomed by the *Jumbe* because the owners appreciated the opportunity to have their stock inspected; they had a wholesome respect for rinderpest and for the measures that had suppressed previous outbreaks in the locality. This was typical of the mutual respect which existed between cattle owners thoughout the whole country and the Veterinary Department. The *Bwana Mganga wa Ngombe* (cow doctor) was their *rafiki* (friend).

During the next three days we inspected 3,500 head of cattle. The grazing areas in the vicinity of the river were now practically bare and the cattle were having to trek further and further afield each day for grass. Despite this, the adult cattle with a few exceptions were still in reasonably good condition. These exceptional individuals had dry, staring coats, were notably thin and almost invariably had enlarged superficial lymph nodes. The enlarged nodes were suggestive of East Coast fever but this was unlikely to be prevalent in such arid surroundings. We had taken along the necessary equipment and reagents for diagnostic microscopy and some haematology. Blood haemoglobin levels were low and smears from the lymph nodes all showed the protozoan parasite *Trypanosoma vivax* so we were able to conclude that the condition was trypanosomiasis rather than East Coast fever which, in any event, would be unlikely to be active during the dry season in such arid conditions. The shortage of grass was driving the herds deeper and deeper into tsetse bush; obviously many cattle were going to die of starvation complicated by trypanosomiasis as the drought progressed.

The cloudless nights were refreshingly cool at Karitu, compared with the extreme dry heat of midday. Our needs for water from the river, firewood and food, in the form of chickens or a sheep, were well catered for by the villagers. After a refreshing bath and a good meal one could wish for no pleasure greater than the tranquillity of sitting for an hour or two before bed at the fire in front of the tent, listening to the night noises, including the murmur of my own chaps' conversation as they relaxed around their own fire. In addition to the ubiquitous shrill chirping of the cicadas, the night noises here included the croaking of frogs at the river's edge, the occasional bark of a jackal and the more persistent howling of nearby hyenas. We were on the edge of well-populated game country; hence the fires which were kept going all night. The hyenas had become aware of the presence of Pup, my miniature dachshund, and several were skulking at a judicious distance beyond the fire, clearly visible in the moonlight. They were obviously determined to get her. The innocent creature, never having seen the like of this before, kept sallying forth yapping to chase them off. The crafty hyenas' strategy was to back off, drawing her further and further out with each sally until it was safe for them to pounce. Fortunately, Pup was an obedient little thing and always responded to my whistle before it was too late. But entertaining though the double act was, there was too much at stake so, before long, Pup was tied up and a few rounds from the shotgun persuaded the evil brutes to push off to a safer distance. How sinister the long, bounding stride of the hyenas looked as they loped away in the pale moonlight. We were indeed seeing life in the raw in a part of Africa where survival of the fittest was all around and so obviously the order of the day and, even more so, of the night.

Our onward journey took us twenty miles to a dried up river of sand, which we misguidedly attempted to cross. With only a few feet to go to the opposite bank the back wheels dug in; we were good and truly stuck and there was nobody but us to get ourselves out. Most lorries in Tanganyika in those days carried an ingeniously simple jack, which consisted of a ratchet embedded in a stout length of timber. The ratchet was cranked upwards by a handle. The rear wheels were jacked up high enough to enable whatever materials were available, such as bushes and palm fronds, to be stuffed under the wheels in order to bind the sand. In those days, before the advent of four-wheel-drives, one could not win; one was either held up by sand rivers in the dry season or swamps and impassable rivers in the wet season. On this occasion, we gained only a foot or two at each attempt and it took us four hours to get onto firm ground at the other side. By then it was almost dark. There is nothing worse than trying to pitch tents after dark so we forged on in the hope of coming to a village but after a few miles our headlights suddenly picked up two huge corrugated iron sheds at the side of the track. It was as surprising as meeting an elephant in Piccadilly Circus. The sheds had apparently been built by the Department of Agriculture for the collection and storage of cotton. In no time the lamps were lit and the Bwana was set up with his table, chair and lonely camp bed in one of the vast sheds. That morning I had shot a Thompson's gazelle so the main course for my candlelight dinner was liver and onions on a bed of rice. The rest of the gang ate and subsequently slept at a discreet distance at the cook's fire at the other end of the vast shed.

As my remit was to examine the cattle along the Manonga and Sibiti Rivers it was necessary for me to stick close to the rivers but after the previous day's experience with the sand river I took no more chances. Therefore, when the necessity arose the lorry took a sweep to the north to find safer crossings while I continued on foot with the Veterinary Guard and one of the Scouts to rendezvous at a pre-arranged spot eight to ten miles further along the river. It was essential to travel as light as possible on these occasions because of the oppressive heat of the day so we carried only a rifle and a shotgun, water bottles, and a jam jar for each of us containing my favourite lunch, namely curried rice liberally laced with hard boiled egg, peas, shredded coconut, and ground nuts. Game was plentiful, particularly in the stretches of tsetse bush through which we travelled and, being on foot, we got close to eland, wildebeest, zebra, kudu, giraffe, Thompson's gazelle, warthogs, bush pigs and, on one occasion a herd of elephants. Of them all, my favourite was the giraffe. I can still see them turning their heads to look at us and then trotting away so gracefully in their inimitable way with their long legs and necks beautifully co-ordinated, giving an impression almost of slow motion. The giraffe, presumably because of its large numbers in the Tanganyika of those days, was the official emblem of the country even to the extent that its head and neck was embossed on the brass buttons of our field service uniforms.

As we progressed eastwards towards Lake Eyasi the effects of the drought became progressively more harrowing as we crossed the Sibiti which was the name given to the vast expanse of plain to the north of that river. For obvious reasons we camped at various points along the course of the river: our need for water and to meet people. There we saw the effects of the drought at their worst because the pressure of the human population and that of their animals returning from further afield to drink had reduced the banks and much of the ground in the immediate vicinity to a covering of white sand. There was no water in the tributaries of the main river, not even waterholes, just the same fine sand. Out on the plain the grass had been grazed to the roots, the earth was cracked, while all the time a strong east wind, punctuated by a succession of whirlwinds, was relentlessly carrying away clouds of fine, powdery dust. Vast quantities of topsoil were being lost. Small herds of cattle, sheep and goats trailed across the shimmering plain pathetically searching for grass roots. Those with young at foot had lost their milk, so calves, lambs and kids that had not already died tried to follow their dams in search of something to eat. As so often in Africa, the situation along the Sibiti River was reminiscent of biblical times. In later years I was reminded of the scene when I came across a passage in Chapter 14 of Jeremiah: 'The ground is cracked because there is no rain in the land, the farmers are dismayed and cover their heads. Even the doe in the field deserts her newborn because there is no grass'.

From time to time a dense cloud of dust on the horizon heralded the approach of large herds of cattle returning from higher ground to the north where there was still some grass, but no water. These herds grazed up there for two or three days and then trekked back to fill their bellies with water. Though the water was life-sustaining they had to live on their fat during the trek. The calves, of course, could not accompany the herd. We continued to look for signs of rinderpest as we had done at Karitu and our other stopping places along the Manonga River. Fortunately our findings were more or less the same; there was no sign of the disease. The few small herds that had remained in the general vicinity of the river were now in very bad condition and many were suffering from trypanosomiasis. The majority of the cattle in the large herds returning from better grazing further afield to drink at the river were still in surprisingly good condition, though a proportion were already in a sorry state. The latter were almost invariably shown to be infected with trypanosomes. The owners quite resignedly accepted what was going on, regarding it as a *shauri la Mungu* (affair of God). When I talked to them they agreed that they all had too many cattle for the available land during the periodic droughts which were, and still are, a feature of the climate of Central Tanganyika. Despite the fact that their social status was governed by the possession of cattle, the more the better, some accepted that the Government should impose drastic culling provided the same proportion of cattle from each herd was taken so that the relative status quo remained the same. If that were done, it would be accepted as a *shauri la Serkali* (affair of the Government).

The losses from starvation must have been devastating during the remainder of the year until the short rains began in November. Sadly, the harmful effects of a severe drought extend long beyond the eventual onset of the next rains. As pointed out in the Department's Annual Report for 1946, droughts of this kind also initiate a vicious circle with long-term effects that can be even more destructive than the immediate death of animals from starvation, loss of condition and the stunted growth of young stock. The herds and flocks are forced into tsetse belts and areas affected with tick-borne diseases and, in the case of cattle, the cows go into prolonged anoestrus and fail to breed, so the calf crop is small in the subsequent year. Furthermore, nature culls the better producers; the law of the survival of the fittest does not in this case safeguard the productivity of the herd. The drying up of the smaller streams and wells leads to massive concentrations of stock within reach of permanent watering points. This creates a spiral of overstocking, denudation of pastures and exclusion of fires because there is not enough grass to get the seasonal flames going in the established areas of bush. This is followed by further encroachment of light bush into the open grazing areas. The tsetse fly moves into the extended areas of bush with the consequent exclusion of stock which, in due course, leads to increased congestion and consequently more erosion of the remaining open range. The countermeasures adopted by the Veterinary and other Departments consisted of encouraging the sale of surplus non-breeding stock; the improvement of marketing facilities and stock routes to the canning factory in Kenya; the provision of more wells and reservoirs; and the selective clearing of bush for the establishment of tsetse-free grazing reserves for use in the dry season. The latter measure was the only practical means of conserving fodder for the dry season because, in those days, the possibility of making hay or silage on range-land was out of the question.

By now we had seen between 30,000 and 40,000 head of cattle. There had been no evidence of serious transmissible diseases, apart from trypanosomiasis. As we drove the next forty miles, to Kimali we followed a rough track into higher ground which became progressively more wooded and cooler with every mile. The shaded, more enclosed sur-roundings of this undulating countryside were delightfully refreshing after the seemingly boundless expanse of the shimmering Sibiti. The discom-fort of our sojourn in that hostile environment made me deeply regret the hardship we inflicted on a group of women whom we took by surprise as we rounded a sharp curve of the track. There they were, in single file, each balancing an obviously heavy load on their heads. As so often happens on such an occasion, they panicked and scurried into the bush at the side of the road and, in doing so, a few of them stumbled and lost their loads. On hitting the ground, the loads split, irretrievably scattering the precious contents - salt - onto the sandy ground. The whole party was frightened and the three unfortunates utterly dismayed. We learnt from the few men who, armed with spears, were accompanying the women that the party had trekked from afar and had crossed the Sibiti to a salt lake where they had spent a harrowing time harvesting the salt. I tried to console the three women with money for the loss of their precious cargo, but for people utterly untouched by consumer society and far removed from shops, a handful of shillings meant little to them. It was salt they were after and now they and their families would have to share their neighbours' stock. The incident was a telling reminder of how utterly dependent *Homo sapiens* is on two simple elements, sodium and chlorine, for the very maintenance of life itself. In extensive areas of Tanganyika, untouched by commerce in those days, man was no better off in this important matter than the herds of game that trek periodically to salt licks, the location of which happen to be known to them through some obscure mechanism.

On arrival at the small village of Kimale we made our way to the rest camp on the nearby stock route. This particular route led all the way from Western Province through the south of Lake Province and onwards through Northern Province to Leibig's canning factory on the Athi River just outside Nairobi. The route was busy at this time of drought with upwards of ten thousand head of cattle passing through each month. This was to prove to be my first significant exposure to the actual working of the stock routes. In Western Province I had only been personally involved in issuing movement permits, hearing the reports of the Veterinary Guards and, while on safari, encountering, from time to time, mobs of cattle trekking through the bush between overnight rest camps. On this occasion, however, I was thrown into an outbreak of foot and mouth disease and, as a result I had an opportunity to see the whole system in action. I was taken by surprise to find a Veterinary Guard at the camp who explained that three days previously eighty head of cattle had arrived at Kimali with three animals showing symptoms of foot and mouth disease. He had retained them in quarantine but, unfortunately, during the next two days three more infected herds comprising a total of 520 cattle had arrived and joined the other eighty in quarantine. On examining the movement permits and questioning the headmen in charge of each mob about the exact location of the rest camp at which symptoms of the infection had first been seen, it was possible to conclude that a fifty mile stretch of the stock route to the west of Kimali was infected. Although there was still reasonable grass cover at the Kimale grazing reserve the 600 cattle now in quarantine would soon lay it bare and force incoming mobs into the surrounding tsetse bush. The mortality from trypanosomiasis would greatly exceed that from foot and mouth disease so, after some hesitation, I lifted the quarantine and left instructions that only infected animals that were unable to walk should be held back. Thereupon, I made my way as quickly as possible to the District Headquarters at Shanwa, some sixty miles to the west, where I telegraphed my report on the foot and mouth disease to Headquarters. I left it to the Director to decide whether or not to close the stock route at an appropriate point. Almost immediately I received a reply and was much relieved to learn that they were satisfied with what I had done. After my long safari through almost trackless bush I marvelled at the efficacy of the low-tech telephone network of simple copper wire that ran along the railway lines and branched out here and there to even the most remote administrative centre.

There were other telegrams and letters awaiting me and it was good to be in contact with the outside world again. A letter from the Acting P.V.O. at Mwanza, Carl Anderson, told me that Micky Norton was at Shinyanga where he was now waiting for further instructions. He emphasised that Micky was my 'baby' now so I sent the lorry to bring him and his entourage up to Maswa, where I too was killing time. When he arrived I was glad to see that he was looking well, despite the fact that he had been having treatment for a varicose ulcer at Shinyanga. He also had the drink under control and we spent a few pleasant days while the job of working out his next itinerary was interspersed with more priceless stories of his earlier life. Before reporting in to Mwanza, I drove him further north to Bumera where he was to pick up porters and patrol an area into which herds of game were streaming from the Serengeti. We had become good friends and as we parted my heart went out to this old man as he was being dumped down in bush, varicose veins and all, so far removed in time and space from his own kith and kin. At least he had the company of his faithful band of camp followers.

My next month in Lake Province was for the most part utterly boring, living out of a suitcase, for a few days at a time, in a tiny room in a grotty hotel in Mwanza. *Mpishi* and Selemani found accommodation somewhere at the back of the building. They too had nothing to do, other than my laundry, so morale deteriorated. It was even a relief to get out across the bone dry, largely treeless terrain of Sukumaland, which I had come to hate, to investigate more reports of cattle dying. Such deaths almost invariably turned out to be cases of trypanosomiasis resulting from drought-stricken herds being pushed deeper and deeper into tsetse bush in search of fodder. A welcome break was initiated by a panic-laden telegram from the District Commissioner at Bukoba, one hundred miles by steamer across Lake Victoria from Mwanza. Bloated carcasses were floating down the Kagera River ten miles from the Uganda border and twenty miles east of the lake shore; was it rinderpest? The huge Kagera River is about 300 miles long and for most of its length forms the frontier between Tanganyika and Rwanda, which was then part of the Belgian Congo. Five miles from its mouth it crosses the Tanganyika border into Uganda where it flows into Lake Victoria. Mpwapwa had been informed and because of the strategic position of the suspected outbreak telegrams had been sent to the Veterinary Departments of Uganda and the Belgian Congo, copied to District Officers of the Provincial Administration to the south and to the Provincial Veterinary Officer of Western Province. The multiplicity of telegrams flying around transmitted the jitters to me so I sent one of my own to the African Veterinary Assistant at Bukoba instructing him to acquire five healthy susceptible yearlings and isolate them as best he could. He was then to inoculate three with blood from one of the carcasses and record the early morning temperatures of the five yearlings pending my arrival.

Carl Anderson jumped at the chance of a trip to Bukoba and decided to come with me. It would be a refreshing change for him to enjoy the cool, moist climate at the other side of the lake after the dry heat of Mwanza and the tedium of being tied to a desk for weeks on end. I was glad to have his company because he and his wife Marjorie had been very kind to me on the various occasions when I returned to Mwanza from my tedious perambulations through Sukumaland. We had become good friends. They were probably in their early fifties but the age difference made no difference to our friendship. Indeed, as far as Marjorie was concerned, it seemed to help because they were childless and it gradually dawned on me that she was taking a motherly interest in me - a little home cooking to take on safari, holes in my precious stockings that had to be darned, and so on. On one of my safaris I had grown a Ronald Colman moustache and on my next visit to their house she took a pained look and all she had to say was "Oh, no!" It was off before the next visit!

By the time we were ready to leave for Bukoba we had missed the weekly steamer so we set off on a 500 mile trip around the south of the lake on good dry-season roads. We did 220 miles on the first day to Kahama in my old territory of Western Province where we stayed the night with the Assistant District Officer, an acquaintance of mine. That sort of hospitality was par for the course in the Tanganyika of those days, particularly on small stations where isolated Europeans were generally hungry for company.

We left Kahama at the crack of dawn and drove 150 miles before lunch to Biharamoulo, the Administrative Headquarters of that District. Most of the journey was through oppressive, largely uninhabited, dense forest. So far we had not had even a glimpse of Lake Victoria which was now fairly close to our right, but some thirty miles after Biharamoulo we gradually emerged into more open grassland and then ground slowly up a long steep hill into Bukoba District. Suddenly, about a thousand feet immediately below us, we saw a vast expanse of the great inland sea stretching brilliantly blue, as far as the eye could see, to the light grey of the distant horizon. All around us were rolling emerald-green hills covered with unbroken carpets of lush grass nourished by the humid air from the lake. In the valleys, banana plantations showed up as deeper shades of green. As we drove the remaining sixty miles across the flatter land, along the shore of the lake towards the town of Bukoba, feathery eucalyptus trees began to line the road. The density of the population seemed to increase as more people appeared on the roadside and, the further we progressed, little villages almost hidden by their plots of banana grew closer and closer together. Here in Bukoba District, as in Uganda not far to the north, the banana was king, the very staff of life, and coffee was the money-spinner. The aridity of the Sabiti with its dust, its wind devils and encroaching starvation, and the monotonous, treeless sweeps of Sukumaland at the other side of the lake were different worlds from Bukoba with its benign climate and its soft, rain-fed verdure.

It was almost dark by the time we reached Bukoba town and found the hotel full, but we were eventually given the keys to an empty bungalow located in a lovely garden close to the lake shore. Next morning I was awakened by Carl squeezing a fresh strawberry into my mouth, a fruit I had not seen for almost two years, but then this was Bukoba! When we located the African Veterinary Assistant the next morning, he informed us that he had examined several carcasses, which had been hauled out of the river, and had seen no lesions suggestive of rinderpest or anything else. So all he had been able to do was to sub-inoculate yearlings as I had requested. So far, none of them had reacted. He tactfully suggested that the District Commissioner had been fussing. We were inclined to agree when we called on this gentleman. With no more carcasses floating past and three more days to go before the next sailing of the steamer to Mwanza there was nothing more to do than enjoy a pleasant drive up river along the road that hugged the Kagera River for fifty miles inland. There was no word along the way about cattle dying. Fifty-two years later, while watching the ghastly pictures on television of human bodies tumbling down the turbulent river from Rwanda during the notorious genocide of 1998 I suddenly realised that I had seen that turbulent river before. I had indeed been there, and as I watched the pictures on the screen of bodies tumbling over and over I was thankful that my job had been merely to search the river for 'lower' animals that had died of natural causes, rather than to witness the results of unspeakable obscenity in such magnificent surroundings.

Over the weekend, we enjoyed the amenities of our lakeside bungalow and the hospitality of the nearby Club. There was an extensive area of long grass along the lakeside between the bungalow and the Club where lots of hippos grazed during the night. We were warned never to get between the hippos and the lake when walking home after dark, even when sober. By Monday morning the inoculated cattle were still showing no reaction so we booked a cabin on the steamer and, with tongue in cheek, thanked the D.C. for a most enjoyable weekend, loaded the lorry that evening and sailed for Mwanza where we docked fifteen hours later. The distance from Bukoba to Manza was twice the distance from Dublin to Holyhead, and just as choppy, reminding one that Lake Victoria is indeed an inland sea.

On my return to Mwanza Carl and Marjorie insisted that I move from the grotty hotel to where they lived, accompanied, of course, by the ever-adaptable Selemani and *Mpishi*. The contrast was unbelievable. I was given the key to the door, to come and go as I liked, and in all other respects I was spoiled rotten. It was unsatisfactory, however, living from day to day waiting for further instructions from Mpwapwa. So, to break the monotony, I shuttled unofficially in my own car between Mwanza and Musoma, also on the Lake shore 160 miles to the north by road and fifty miles south of the Kenya border. My idea was to lend a hand to Mac, who in addition was great fun. Another attraction, however, was two pretty nursing sisters at the local hospital with no other bachelors for miles around.

Eventually, my instructions came through to Mwanza. I was to return to Musoma to pick up a lorry from Mac and then proceed through the Serengeti National Park to the famous Ngorogoro Crater, which had the greatest concentration of game in the world, and from there to Mbulu a hundred miles south on the Masai Steppe. I was to spend three weeks on that leg of the journey, the whole point of which was to familiarise myself with the Masai and at the same time to keep an eye open for disease in game. From Mbulu I was to head north to Arusha where I was to report to the Provincial Veterinary Officer who would arrange a tour of European farms in the Arusha and Moshi Districts, on the lower slopes of Mounts Meru and Kilimanjaro, respectively. The object of that tour was to study the veterinary problems occurring on European-owned farms. Looking back, the whole safari sounded as exciting as winning a fantastic holiday on one of today's TV quiz shows! There was a bonus at the end of the memo. I was to send surplus heavy loads and the car by train from Mwanza to Mpwapwa, which I interpreted as indicating that I was going back to the laboratory, probably for the remainder of my tour; and Micky Norton, who was now referred to by Carl and Marjorie as my heavenly twin, was to accompany me to the edge of the Serengeti!

It was going to be cold country from Ngorogoro onwards, so before parting with my heavy loads I took great pleasure in extracting a tweed jacket, sweater, riding breeches and blankets for the journey. The extraction of the blankets brought a frown to Selemani's face but he cheered up when I assured him that I would be buying the same for him. *Mpishi* had found the shiftless life of the past two months hard going and wanted nothing more than to get back to a settled life in Tabora so his resignation was accepted with genuine regret all round. His departure presented a problem but the resourceful Selemani told me not to worry; he knew of a cook in Musoma who was looking for a job.

Jack Holloway happened to be on safari in Lake Province so, having seen the cook and my own car safely on the train, I hitched a lift in his lorry to Musoma. Micky Norton had not materialised from bush by then so it was arranged that he would travel with his entourage from Mwanza to Musoma by the lake steamer while I was preparing the safari from there. Fortunately, the only vehicle that Mac could spare was out in bush and it took some days to get it back to Musoma. This gave me time to recruit Jackson Bwire who turned out to be another excellent cook and, above all, utterly reliable and honest. He remained with me for the rest of my time in Tanganyika.

On the eve of my departure from Musoma, Mac and I had dinner with the nursing sisters and afterwards we sat for a while on an Arab *dhow* at the bottom of the garden. It was a perfect setting in which to say good-bye: a boat, rolling gently on the swell; and a full moon rising above the horizon, slowly becoming visible through the papyrus grass at the margin of the lake. As it rose higher in the sky the moon shed a path of silver across the lake until it suddenly disappeared behind a low-lying bank of thundercloud. Once more all was darkness, the spell was broken and we again became conscious of croaking frogs, the eerie howling of a hyena in the distance and the constant lapping of the water. Had it not been for the sudden intervention of the dark cloud and the presence of Mac and his companion, I do believe I might well have popped the question! We did not meet again for some ten years. By then we were both happily married, so I refrained from asking my friend whether she too remembered that thundercloud.

Next morning, as Micky Norton and I set off with our combined entourage in an over-loaded lorry, I had no idea of the extent to which I was about to be educated further in the extraordinary physical, biological and social diversity of this wonderful country, Tanganyika in terms of the topography of its vast plains and towering mountains; its climatic and botanical variations; its differing agricultural and social systems; and the variations in the concentrations of its vast stock of feral animals and the diversity of their specific components. At that stage I was unaware that my travels, which during the past three months had taken me from the parched Sibiti Plains through the treeless expanses of Sukumaland and from there to the rain-fed freshness of Bukoba, were to take me beyond Moshi at the foot of snow-capped Kilimanjaro right down to the humid, palm-lined shores of the Indian Ocean at Tanga.

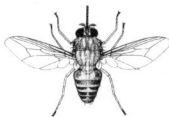

CHAPTER EIGHTEEN

Across the Serengeti

On safari with Micky Norton across the Serengeti. Reflections on the ancient origins of man and the interdependence of all life forms - in proximity to the Olduvai Gorge. Depression on Ngorogoro Crater. Slow progress through inhospitable terrain - stuck in the mud.

The Ford lorry I had borrowed was irreversibly fitted with a device, called a governor, preventing it from exceeding thirty miles per hour, even when dashing at full throttle in the hope of crossing sand or mud at the first shot. That alone augured ill for the journey. Real trouble, however, was assured by the fact that as we left Musoma the lorry was loaded to the gunnels. The load included water and petrol drums, uniform cases full of bedding and clothes, food for a few weeks, cooks' boxes, tents, baths for both Micky and myself; plus shovels and sheets of corrugated iron for getting through. If that were not enough the whole lot was topped off with Selemani and Jackson, a Veterinary Guard, Micky's servants who were armed to the teeth, his Game Scout (also armed), the driver, his turney boy, and the inevitable, uninvited passengers who sneaked aboard as soon as we moved off.

The rains were early that year in Musoma District and the roads were already in bad condition. Consequently, we covered only thirty-six miles that day and did not reach Ikisu until after nightfall. We stayed in a grotty rest house that we were glad to leave at the crack of dawn. That day our aim was to travel eighty miles to drier country at Benagi where, according to Micky, there was an excellent rest house with running water and a bathroom. The area was famous for its lions and the house had been used before the war by royalty, film stars and other wealthy visitors. The journey turned out to be appalling with the lorry bogging down on several occasions up to the axles in mud, wheels spinning helplessly. The routine then saw everybody out (except Micky), unloading, digging, road-making with bush poles and corrugated iron, pushing and eventually re-loading. It was some compensation, as we moved into drier country, to see large herds of hartebeest, zebra, wildebeest, Thompson's gazelle, some impala, a few giraffe and wild pig. The antelope in particular were remarkably tame. Eventually darkness fell and by 9 p.m., when we thought we were in striking distance of our goal, we became bogged down again. Everyone was jaded but Micky, despite his 70 years, was determined that we should have one last go at digging out rather than trying to pitch a tent in the dark and sleeping out in lion country. Almost immediately after re-loading the lorry, for what proved to be the last time, the headlights picked up the rest house. Within fifteen minutes the table was laid and Micky and I were listening to the news on the radio from London! When I awoke next morning to find the sun high in the heavens Micky and the boys were all excited about the lions that had been roaring during the night. I had not heard a thing! The following nights were disturbed for all of us by the almost continuous roaring of the lions down at the near-by stream. It was even more sobering to hear from time to time one, or perhaps more, growling right outside the house. On one occasion even the pragmatic Mickey sat bolt upright in his bed and muttered, 'Jazus, they're close!'

Apart from that, Benagi was indeed an enjoyable stopping place situated almost 5,000 feet above sea level and, therefore, pleasantly cool. The rest house was every bit as comfortable as Micky had described, with a proper bathroom and a supply of piped water from a gently flowing stream nearby. It was odd to find a suburban bungalow, as one might describe it with a little stretch of the imagination, away out on the Serengeti with a radio on the veranda blaring out 'Music While You Work' direct from London! All this with herds of antelope, zebra, wildebeest and other species of game clearly visible only a few hundred yards away. The place had stood practically idle for the past five or six years occupied for most of the time only by the ghosts of royalty and other celebrities. We had a good excuse to stay a while at Benagi as it had been arranged that porters for Micky's safari to the south would meet us here. Furthermore, one of my terms of reference was to look for rinderpest in game, so why not start here? We enjoyed ourselves for a few days cruising around and getting as close as possible to game, at the same time keeping an eye open for vultures circling in the distance. They could be relied upon to spot carcasses for miles around. The country was typical of my preconceived conception of Africa - rolling grassland studded with flat-topped Acacia trees and the occasional hill here and there. It was a happy time.

During my perambulations I came across an abandoned gold mine at Kilimafedha which means 'hill money' or, loosely, 'hill of gold'. The unprotected open shafts, some 200 feet deep, were surrounded by rusty machinery and heaps of tailings. In a few of the rocks I picked through, I saw tiny grains of what appeared to be gold. It was exciting. The winding gantry was still intact above one of the shafts and when I climbed to the top there was a magnificent view of the surrounding country almost up to the Kenya border some forty miles away. The contrast between the vast sweep of virgin territory, unsullied by any sign of human habitation, and the ghost town appearance of the scarred patch now far below my feet, pocked as it was with the crumbling walls of roofless houses, mangled sheets of corrugated iron groaning in the wind, rusting machinery and other debris, was a depressing reminder of man's rapacious greed. It was good to return from the loneliness of Kilimafedha to the buzz at Benagi where Micky's porters had arrived. There was Micky, roaring like a bull, as he supervised the division of his gear and supplies into the regulation head loads of fifty pounds per man. The following day I went out with the Game Department's Game Ranger, who was stationed at Benagi, to shoot a zebra for the pot, which now had to provide for twenty porters as well as ourselves. Despite a complete ban on the killing of any living creature in the Serengeti National Park it was permissible for a vet to shoot any animal he wished, provided disease was suspected. Needless to say, it was also a helpful precaution when shooting for the pot to take the Game Department's Game Ranger along to share the kill! On our return to the house there was a chorus of many 'Ah! Assanti sanas' ('thank you very much') from the porters when they discovered that I had shot no less than a zebra. That night the lions were kept at bay by the dancing and singing which went on into the small hours in the flickering light of a huge fire.

During our time at Benagi Micky and I were more relaxed in each other's company than we had ever been. The evenings passed pleasantly listening to the radio and from time to time to more of his bizarre stories covering the past fifty years in Africa. He had been off the bottle for over two months now and he explained that even in the old days he seldom took more than a bottle or two of whisky on safari in case he might become utterly addicted. Nevertheless, after a few months in bush a point was inevitably reached when he just had to make a beeline for 'the nearest hotel, to the marble-topped tables, the long-necked bottles and a week's oblivion'. When he was so sick that he could drink no more his boys took him out of town to camp for a week or so until he was better. He then disappeared in search of his elephants, feeling a new man, far beyond the arms of the law. He reckoned that drink is the worst illness of all - malaria is nothing in comparison.

On the night before we parted he confided in me that he had two sisters still in Dublin. I urged him to let me find out if they were still alive and, with the naivety of youth, I felt that I had almost persuaded him to take a last trip home to see them before it was too late. Next morning Micky was subdued and did not seem to relish the prospect of striking off on his own. He had obviously enjoyed the company but said little as we parted. Clearly, we both felt our friendship had developed wonderfully well since I had first heard that this countryman of mine was about to burn down a lonely mission station in the depths of Tabora District for the want of a bottle of whisky. That meant nothing now; we had both bridged the age barrier. Perhaps it was Micky who had come of age and I who had matured a little. We had come together, not as father and son - just pals. Several weeks later at Tanga, I received a sad letter from Carl Anderson at Mwanza. Micky had been brought in to hospital at Mwanza with gastric haemorrhage and died peacefully a few days later. As was the custom, the Public Works Department acted as undertakers and provided a lorry for the purpose. As the lorry left the hospital, with the coffin draped in the Union Jack, Micky's camp followers climbed aboard and sat on the coffin for the procession to the cemetery. It was a fitting tribute to an old man who had spent the best years of his life with a private army that had fol-lowed him faithfully through those parts of Portuguese East Africa and Tanganyika where they and their elephants were beyond the reach of the law. I wondered if he would have preferred the green, white and orange Tricolour to the Union Jack for his last safari. Perhaps not; after all, at the end of his days he actually *was* a member of His Majesty's Colonial Service.

The trip across the Serengeti, while relatively uneventful as far as Ngorogoro, was notable for the vast expanses of open grassland, dotted with flat-topped Acacia and stretching for as far as the eye could see. The track grew fainter and petered out from time to time into unbroken ground. That was disturbing. It was comforting, however, to learn from the driver who had passed this way before that the track ran more or less eastwards from one hillock to another in the general direction of Ngorogoro. If one lost the track one could rely on picking it up again on the approach to the next hill. Game was present in such numbers that the only way in which one could ascertain whether or not there was disease in the area was to look out for vultures hovering over a dying animal or a recent kill. During the course of the hundred mile journey from Benagi to the Crater we met no fellow humans other than a group of Masai on the move with their cattle. While we chatted pleasantly they assured us that they had not seen any sign of rinderpest during their travels. The Masai knew what they were talking about and could always be relied upon in such matters.

On the afternoon of our last day on the Serengeti we were relieved to have managed, without incident, to cross a treacherous tract of lava dust that was practically devoid of game and were again driving through extensive open savannah with an increasing amount of tree cover. Late afternoon is a delightful time for such a drive. The scenery takes on more varied, gentler colours after the harsh sunshine of midday and the herds of antelopes and other game, many of which have been less obvious during the heat of the day, emerge from the limited shade and are seen grazing in even greater numbers. I rolled back the canvas cover on top of the lorry and seated myself on the loads for this special time.

As we sped along the rising ground on our approach to Ngorogoro I was deeply conscious of how unspoiled the scene was with its huge population of game animals, composed of such a multiplicity of species, and the complete absence of human beings. With my memories of the bare, eroded tracts of Central Province and the drought-stricken, over-populated Sibiti Plains fresh in my mind I felt I was looking at country which had remained unchanged in the safe hands of Mother Nature over countless centuries, perhaps millennia. Successive generations of the animals which we were now passing, and other species presently unseen, had been giving birth here over the ages and suckling their young. Those that survived had been growing to maturity, then breeding at the appointed times, giving birth to their young and in their own turn dying to make room for succeeding generations. Each species played its own particular part in maintaining the delicate balance between the flora and the fauna on this expanse of savannah that sustained them all. The various species of antelopes and other herbivores which grazed the pasture exclusively, and those that also browsed on bush and trees, maintained the balance between the pasture and its tree cover. Of equal importance was the fact that all the herbivores present, in such numbers and in such a variety of species, had one characteristic in common; they themselves were sustained by their ability to convert cellulose into compact, high-energy foodstuff, namely meat, on which all the species of carnivores were completely dependent. In return, their carnivorous predators restricted the growth of the populations on which they preyed and thereby played their part in preserving the integrity of the soil. Finally, this very soil fed the greenery whose chlorophyll trapped the energy from the sun on which the whole cycle depended.

As I feasted my eyes on the tranquillity of this vast Garden of Eden, stretching for as far as the eye could see, it was hard to accept that the evolution of this and all other ecosystems had arisen, as many believed, from primeval chemical reactions that created the first sparks of life. It was even more difficult to accept that such sparks had eventually led to the evolution of *Homo sapiens* and his ability, not only to see, but also to be moved emotionally by the beauty of the scene. At the time I passed that way, I had no idea that I was actually within a stone's throw of the Olduvai Gorge - indeed I had not even heard of its existence. Years later I learnt that the treasures hidden in the gorge were first brought to the attention of the world of science by a German lepidopterist who passed that way, just before the First World War, in search of rare species of butterflies. During his search serendipity intervened and he found that the gorge was a virtual museum for relics of extinct, prehistoric creatures such as short-necked giraffes, three-toed members of the equidae and hippopotamuses with eyes like periscopes. In 1931 the subsequently famous palaeontologist, L.S. Leakey, began his life work in the gorge and he and his wife Mary unearthed stone tools and the skull of an early hominid which carbondating showed to be almost two million years old. Perhaps my drowsy meditation had been prompted by something in the air as I passed that way.

With about twenty-five miles to go to the edge of the crater, still some 3,000 feet above us, we started our tortuous climb at a snail's pace. Though the light was beginning to fade the slow pace, coupled with the twisting and turning of the road, gave us magnificent views of the vast plains and mountains that we were leaving behind. As we climbed progressively higher the vegetation became more lush and the atmosphere so damp and cold that I was soon forced into the relative warmth of the cab, leaving the unfortunate Africans swathed in blankets on the back of the lorry. Long after darkness had fallen the headlights picked up a noticeboard through the mist which read 'Ngorogoro Rest Camp two miles'. To my great relief the camp turned out to be a number of substantial log cabins with plenty of room for us all but this did nothing to raise the spirits of the boys who were now so miserable from cold that they could hardly think properly. Admittedly, the contrast between the heat on the bone dry larva dust at midday and the piercing cold at the crater edge only hours later was horrendous. Fortunately, the cabins were well stocked with firewood so the first job was to light the fires. As soon as the flames started crackling up the chimney I found myself automatically standing legs apart with my back to the fire; I had not needed to air myself like that since leaving England two years previously. Miraculously, a meal of some sort appeared and after that I retired to the luxury of four blankets and enjoyed the long-forgotten experience of gradually edging my feet down between two cold sheets.

I awoke with a sense of expectancy and as I came to I realised that this was due to the fact that I was to see, or so I thought, the crater for the first time. Even so, my nose was so cold that I lay wallowing in the luxury of the warmth between the sheets until Selemani appeared with a cup of tea, looking the picture of misery and even more droopy than ever swathed in layers of blankets trailing down to his feet. He did, however, manage to grin and said 'Auch, shocking cold! What sort of place is this

Ngorogoro?' When I eventually looked out there was nothing to be seen but thick fog so I sat huddled over the fire for most of the morning until there was a brief break in the clouds. This revealed that we were right on the crater's edge looking down to its floor about one or two thousand feet below. It stretched for more than twenty miles across to the opposite wall, for all the world like a great saucer. The general greyness of our surroundings, the overhanging mist, the moss-covered tree trunks, the silence and loneliness of the whole place was depressing. I forced myself to go for a stroll and through the mist I got a glimpse of a herd of black cattle grazing in a hollow nearby. I scrambled down in the hope of having a chat with some Masai but to my horror I realised I was almost into a herd of buffalo, some of the most dangerous animals to meet in such circumstances.

By now my travelling companions were thoroughly demoralised, skulking around with glum faces. The driver and Selemani were delegated to approach me. Selemani in his characteristic posture for such occasions - shoulders hunched, turning his head first to the right and then to the left to avoid looking me straight in the eyes - explained that they were all very ill and were shivering as if they had malaria, but they knew they were not sick, it was just the cold, when were we going? I agreed and added, 'First thing tomorrow'.

My instructions were to go to a place called Kakesio, some thirty miles south-west near Lake Eyasi within striking distance of the dreaded, drought-stricken Sibiti Plains, to talk to a settlement of the Masai in the vicinity. That involved getting down off the mountain to the tiny village of Endulen and proceeding from there to Kakesio. The road down from the crater, which was soaked by the almost uninterrupted cloud cover, consisted of a grass bank that had been built up with soil from the verge, leaving a ditch at each side. There were two wheel tracks on the top of the bank which were bare of grass, wet and sticky. At the first incline the lorry, with its speed limited by the governor, began to falter and slithered dangerously close to the edge of the bank. Fortunately, we stopped just in time and fitted chains to the rear wheels. From there on, with much stopping, lightening of loads and pushing, we managed to reach the nearby branch road which wound downhill to emerge from the clouds. Within a few miles, with the chains off, a cloud of dust rose up behind us as we sped into the village of Endulen. We had not seen a *duka* since we left Musoma and when we spotted one we stopped to find that it had a few bags of flour and sugar, which enabled us to replenish our supplies - we were back in the consumer society!

Thirteen miles further on we pitched our tents at Kakesio which we found was nothing more than a dilapidated Somali *duka* that seemed to exist for nothing more than buying a hide or two from the self-sufficient Masai in return for a few ounces of tea, salt or an occasional blanket. There were two Masai *bomas* nearby. Nevertheless, it was a lonely place. Word had got around that a '*Bwana Mganga wa Ngombe* (a vet or, literally, a 'Bwana doctor of cattle') had arrived, and early next morning a group of Masai called to greet me. After the formal handshakes, with one hand behind the back to convey that one was unarmed, they asked me for news of the safari and in accordance with protocol I enquired about the *habari za hapa* (news of here). Having assured me that there was no rinderpest in the area they began to tell me about the diseases that affected their cattle from time to time. During their description of the symptoms of a particular disease I began to chip in as soon as I reckoned precisely what it was and added a few more symptoms. My interruptions provoked profound astonishment accompanied by exclamations of, '*Aah! Kweli; ndio, kweli kabisa*' (loosely, 'True! Yes absolutely true'). Their joy was complete when I produced a book and showed them a photograph of one of the diseases we had been discussing. We had become blood brothers - without a drop of blood having been drawn! Their good humour was admirable considering that the rain we had encountered at Musoma and on the crater had not reached as far as Kakesio and the surrounding area was still drought-stricken. There was abundant water in the stream, which was fed from the mountain, but the ground was bare, so emaciated cattle were watered every second or third day and then trekked back to areas not yet denuded of grass. The dung of one moribund heifer that I examined was composed of undigested Acacia seeds and sand.

Our onward journey from Kakesio was to take us to Arusha via Oldeani but this meant returning again to the wretched crater, so we holed up near Endulen for a couple of days to wash our clothes and bake bread. The site we chose beside a bubbling brook seemed perfect. After dark it turned out to be a haunt for a pack of hyenas that loped around our tents all night. The howling of hyenas, especially when a whole pack is involved, is diabolical and can be quite unnerving when one is wakened from fitful sleep by grunts and rustling nearby. Consequently, I had confined Pup in the cab of the lorry and gone to bed with my shotgun within reach. I was subsequently relieved to learn that I was not the only one with the wobbles when the driver, looking rather shamefaced, woke me up to ask for some cartridges for his gun and told me that he and his pals had left their tent for the sanctuary of the lorry!

After two days of regular meals we set off for Oldeani at the crack of dawn, refreshed, despite the broken nights. Our spirits were high as our target was the civilisation of Oldeani, which we hoped to reach that night. It became important to do so because we had agreed to take a sick Masai *moran*, who appeared to be suffering from pneumonia, and his companion to hospital at Oldeani without delay. What a vain hope it turned out to be! We retraced our steps almost to the rest camp at the crater and turned right for Oldeani, with eighteen miles to go. The road over the mountain was even worse than it had been previously. Before long we lost momentum and with the back wheels spinning from side to side the engine cut out and we came to rest with one wheel on the very edge of the ditch. (See illust.) The only thing to do was to jack up the back wheels as best we could, dig down into the side of the bank for dry soil with which to build a new bit of road under the wheels, and repeat the process until the back of the lorry was on the original level. We then fitted chains to the rear wheels, which we should have done before, and laid a track of dry soil for some twenty yards in front of the lorry. Finally, after much pushing, she moved off gingerly while we held our breath and watched her climb slowly to the top of the hill. Thereafter, there was a succession of hills and hollows on several of which we had to repeat the wretched process over and over again. The slow pace and general misery of the journey convinced me that a lorry in these circumstances was a liability; we would willingly have pushed the wretched vehicle into the nearest ravine had we been able to get our hands on Micky Norton's porters for a good old-fashioned walking safari.

By nightfall we had covered only four miles. By then we were cold, wet, covered in mud and utterly dispirited. All that had kept us going was the hope that each stop would prove to be the last and that we would soon emerge from the clouds onto dry ground again. There was no point, however, in trying to strike camp because everything was soaking wet, there was no dry firewood and we were all worn out. Consequently, we went on with fingers crossed for another mile until one of the chains broke loose and began to lash the chassis with an almighty clamour. It was now pouring rain so most of the boys stayed put under the leaking canopy on the back of the lorry while the driver and his turney boy climbed under the chassis to fix the chain. I stayed in the cab with a foot on the brake to immobilise the wheel while he worked away. He was a long time on the job and I was suddenly aroused from a daydream by somebody shouting. I jumped down, now wide awake, to find the turney boy trying to haul the driver out from under the lorry. The driver had left the engine running to save the battery and had inhaled the exhaust fumes. We dragged his limp body into the beam of the headlights and found he was almost unconscious and barely breathing. In those days I had never even heard of mouth-to-mouth resuscitation so all I could do was to squat across his stomach and pump his chest as best I could. That brought a series of groans and after what seemed an age he gradually got back to normal breathing. When he regained his wits we lifted him to his feet and he staggered a few paces, then turned round to stare at us. It was an eerie sight in the misty glare of the headlights. The rest of the party stood wide-eyed. One of them murmured 'Ah Shatani, Shatani – there's a devil in him now'. We rummaged in the loads to find a few dry blankets to wrap him in before settling him down in the back of the lorry.

The chain was still off, buried in mud, and with the rain belting down we were stuck good and proper; we could neither move on nor even attempt to pitch the tents. All we could do was to throw off most of the loads to clear sleeping space for the boys and make the pneumonic Masai and the driver more comfortable for the night. It was too wet even to attempt to find food so I left the boys to their own devices while I climbed into the cab and curled up with a very wet Pup at my feet. It was too cold, however, to sleep for any length of time and during one of my many waking moments I found a six-month-old copy of the *Irish Times Pictorial* and re-read, of all things, a tourist's description of a trip on horseback through the famous Gap of Dunloe in a rain storm! It was a very long night! It was hard to know when the dawn came, it did not actually break, it just changed gradually from pitch dark to a misty grey, revealing that we were enveloped in dense fog. My exit from the cab elicited no response from the back of the lorry. When I went to enquire about the driver I found everybody, other than the driver and the pneumonic Masai sitting up, utterly dispirited. There seemed no point in trying to rouse them so I set off on a long walk in the direction of Oldeani and found that the road was much worse than I had dared to hope. Still, the exercise got the blood circulating and I felt a new man as I retraced my steps purposefully back to the lorry. Nevertheless, my resolve to get us out of there weakened a little when I reached the brow of the hill and viewed the depressing sight of the lorry standing there in the hollow surrounded by the loads scattered higgledy-piggledy in the mud. There was no response from the boys. They were still shivering under the oozing canopy of the lorry.

The turning point was my finding a box of tinned food brought along for just such an emergency. Generous helpings of tinned sausages, fish, and spam improved the morale a little. One of the company was dispatched, armed with my shotgun, in the direction of Oldeani in search of assistance while two of us got down on hands and knees under the lorry in the oozy mud where we set to work on the chains until they were back on the wheel, tied and double tied with stout wire. Meanwhile, the others applied themselves digging for dry soil to put under the wheels and in front of the lorry. We took our time; it was essential that our first attempt should succeed, even for a few yards. Before we were quite ready to start the engine, three wonderful things happened almost simultaneously. The mist cleared, the sun burst through and our messenger appeared over the brow of the hill, actually jogging, with a band of happy, well-fed labourers from a PWD (Public Works Department) camp further along the road. After light-hearted greetings and a bit of bantering the merry reinforcements applied themselves energetically to the back of the lorry. Everybody pushed while I let the clutch out gingerly. The wheels skidded from side to side for a moment then got their grip and the lorry climbed slowly to the top of the hill. The spell was broken. The scattered loads were retrieved from the bottom of the hill and everybody applied himself cheerfully to the job of loading while I attended to the pneumonic Masai and the driver.

The driver was, of course, still out of the game so I had to drive. Although I seldom exceeded 5 m.p.h. the lorry periodically got out of control, ending up in the ditch. Our reinforcements stuck with us and the digging-out became almost a happy routine. We emerged eventually from the dank forest and there, stretching for miles below us, were the huge smiling fields of the European farms at Oldeani. At that point we parted with our PWD friends who returned happily to their misty eyrie while we set off on a slithering descent to dry ground. There we removed the chains before spinning along with the driver and the Masai to the hospital. Even the Masai seemed to be none the worse for his night on the mountain although the driver was still a bit groggy when we left him there to be checked out. The next stop on the way to the comfort of the rest house was a stop at the *dukas* where, amongst other good things, I saw and bought a slab of Nestle's milk chocolate - the first I had seen since before the war!

Oldeani was a pleasantly warm place in marked contrast to the cold, dank atmosphere of the crater and the arid heat of Kakesio. It was more of a town than a village with its hospital, rest house, several *dukas*, a garage, and there were a number of Europeans around as the area had been fairly intensively settled by Germans before the war. Most of them had been interned as 'enemy aliens' and the management of their farms, with extensive coffee plantations and wheat, had been run by the Custodian of Enemy Property since 1939.

Having completed our safari across the Serengeti, repaired the lorry, rested the driver and bought fuel and other provisions for the return journey it was time to dispatch the party back to Musoma. After the trials and tribulations we had shared on the safari the parting was rather touching with full ceremonial handshaking and, in the case of the Veterinary Guard, a final formal salute with an extra firm stamp of the feet. As soon as they were on their way Selemani, Jackson and I were left standing there, perhaps feeling a little lonely after the last wave. Selemani broke the spell by confiding in me that they thought I was an OK Bwana because I had helped to carry loads, push the lorry, got *chafua sana* (very dirty) fixing chains and shooting meat for them. In return, they were all praying that I would soon become *Acting* Director of Veterinary Services. I was not put out by their reluctance to have me promoted straight away to the substantive post. After all, I was still too young for that!

CHAPTER NINETEEN

Arusha, Kiliminjaro and the Coast

A visit to pleasant Arusha but bad news from home. Restful time at the foot of Kilimanjaro. New responsibilities in Tanga. Converting an air base into a dairy farm. Controlling East Coast Fever on the farm. Romance of ships passing in the night - twice!

Later that day, we jumped a lorry and arrived at Arusha where we found Brian Sheriff' at whose house I was to stay. Brian, a twenty-three year old recently arrived Veterinary Officer, had qualified two years after me at Dublin so it was a great Irish reunion with reminiscing and exchange of news over dinner and into the small hours. His short experience of Tanganyika had been very different from mine, having been posted to Arusha as assistant to the Provincial Veterinary Officer of Northern Province. The general environment of Arusha District exemplified the diversity of the climatic and social conditions to be found in Tanganyika. The town itself was remarkably beautiful, placed as it is against the backdrop of Mount Meru, a wonderfully conical mountain almost 15,000 feet above sea level. Situated on the slopes of the mountain Arusha, and the surrounding country, is quite cold. During the colder months one is inclined to wear a tweed jacket and indoors wood fires are generally lit in the evenings. Prior to the First World War, the temperate climate had attracted many Germans to settle in the highlands of northern Tanganyika bordering the equally high ground of the Kenya Plateau. Between the wars most of the alienated land had been acquired by a variety of Europeans (mainly British and Greeks), some Boers from South Africa and Indians. A proportion of the

British types were professional farmers, as were the Boers. Being dependent for their livelihoods on farming they took their vocations seriously
and contributed much to the community. On the other hand, a goodly
number of the British were either the younger sons of English aristocratic
families or others with private means who were attracted by the congenial
climate and a more frivolous lifestyle than they could afford or get away
with at home. The cash flow generated by the expatriate society supported a refreshing number of well-stocked shops, two fine hotels and
other amenities. Next morning, the short journey through the bustling
town on our way to the Provincial Veterinary Office was an exciting
experience after the last two years in what, to me, was the real Africa.

My brief euphoria evaporated when, rifling through a pile of
accumulated mail, I opened the first letter from home. It broke the news
gently that my youngest sister, Anna, had been struck down with tuberculosis, the dread disease which at that time was rampant among young
people in Ireland. It was particularly hard as it was she, my harum-scarum
sister, who had propped me up on the saddle of her bike every Saturday
morning, before my legs were long enough to reach the pedals, and then
stood on them herself and propelled the pair of us zigzagging at high
speed down the hill to the consternation of neighbours. The purpose of
the expedition was to spend our Saturday's penny. A penny was a lot of
money in those days - a ha'penny could buy eight aniseed balls, so it was
a serious business; one had to visit more than one shop! Further down the
pile of letters there were others from most members of the family assuring
me that it was a mild case, not to worry and that she was already making
good progress. Nevertheless, I knew them all too well to be impressed.

Subsequently, however, they were as surprised as I was at the
progress she made during the next two years with nothing more than bed
rest, fresh air and almost forced feeding on a rich diet, since it was long
before the advent of chemotherapy. At the end of the two years she was
discharged and I had the pleasure of sending her on her way from the
British Airways terminal building in Victoria, London to Burma where
she began her married life shuttling to and fro from Rangoon to the
Persian Gulf as the Captain's wife on the flagship of the Burma Oil
Company - still game for anything!

Brian was an excellent host and my first week with him was one long laugh from morning to night. It was not only refreshing after the solitude and discomfort of the past weeks, it was also surprising because my memory of him as my junior by two years at college was of a quiet, serious young man who was much sought after as a church organist. His more relaxed attitude to life may have been brought about by the invigorating surroundings in which he found himself, including the friendships he had made during the course of his work with the more zany members of the settler community. His work in Arusha was so different from what I had experienced elsewhere in Tanganyika. Here in Arusha he was essentially a general practitioner providing a clinical service for the European farmers. I well remember assisting him with the castration of a stallion that had been acquired by the rather dotty wife of one of the more frivolous settlers who did not know one end of a horse from the other. In those days, castration was a rather spectacular performance, involving the casting of the horse with ropes and then anaesthetizing it with chloroform. Some of their equally zany friends had been invited along to see the operation and all were so impressed that a lunch party broke out, after several celebratory rounds of Pimm's and pink gins, and went on for the rest of the afternoon. Life seemed to be one long holiday compared with that of a country practitioner at home!

Arusha was also notable as the terminus of the Northern Railway that ran to Moshi and then south-east to Tanga, some 200 miles away on the Indian Ocean. After my hectic week in Arusha, Brian put me on the train for Moshi where I was to spend two weeks with the Livestock Officer in charge of that area, visiting estates on the foothills of Kilimanjaro and attending to any veterinary problems that needed attention. As things turned out there was really nothing to be done other than to enjoy myself driving around the beautiful country on the slopes of Kilimanjaro. I stayed in the Lion Cub Hotel, a charming little hotel at the foot of Kilimanjaro. My lasting memory of the Lion Cub is the sense of well-being I experienced every night as I strolled across the well-kept garden after an excellent dinner and paused, before going into my own hut, to look up at the magnificent snow-capped mountain, bathed in moonlight and towering up to more than 19,000 feet almost immediately behind the hotel, or so it seemed. Equally pleasant is the memory of the well-preserved, middle-aged lady who had taken it upon herself to teach me the tango over dinner in those exotic surroundings. What a waste of time the nights out on the Crater had been!

After only a few days, the idyllic interlude was abruptly ended by a telegram that informed me that the Director had arrived at Arusha and wanted to see me immediately. Bertie was the sort of man who, in such circumstances, always made you wonder what you had done wrong. He was very courteous, however, as he enquired about my experiences over the past ten months. Then he broke the news. I was to leave for Tanga the next day. Hugh Newlands, the Provincial Veterinary Officer, had been ill for some time and had just been flown to Dar for an appendectomy. He would be off duty for at least a month, so I was to take over the Province. It was not a large Province but the big thing at that moment was that the Government was in the process of taking over a Royal Navy Air Base that was to be developed as a dairy farm for the supply of fresh milk to Tanga. For some reason, it was given a high priority by Government so the Veterinary Department had been allocated considerable funds to do the conversion job and there was much pressure from Dar to get things moving. Consequently, a herd of seventy-five high grade (that is, cross-bred), in-calf heifers had arrived from Kenya three weeks previously, even before proper buildings had been erected. Such animals were highly susceptible to East Coast fever and already there had been two or three mortalities. Bertie Lowe's parting words to me were, 'Now don't forget, no more animals are to die'.

The sun was setting next evening as the train pulled into Moshi and there, standing on the platform, was my dancing partner from the Lion Cub Hotel. I must admit I was somewhat disappointed when she explained that she was not travelling herself; she was merely sending her companion Ruth, a stunning young redhead, on her way. 'Great, I'll settle for that', I said to myself, as I helped the young lady aboard. As I fully intended, we met again in the dining car for dinner and chatted the night away until the train eventually ground to a halt at a wayside station. I was astonished when I saw Neil Reid, the Senior Veterinary Officer from Mpwapwa whom I greatly respected, emerging from the darkness to tap on the window of the dining car. After a rather garbled introduction - I still was unsure of my new friend's surname - Ruth tactfully withdrew to her sleeping compartment. Neil, who had just come up from Tanga, had learnt that I was on the train so he took the opportunity to fill me in hurriedly on the details of the dairy project. On arrival at Tanga next morning, after waiting for Ruth to get off the train, I was informed by the Guard that she had left the train at Korogwe, some forty miles up the line. Dammit, I did not even know her whereabouts, far less her full name - my dream of Tanga as a Garden of Eden ended abruptly.

The good thing about Tanga was that I had been booked into the best hotel, a very good one with only one disadvantage; it was next door to an Indian cinema that operated well into the night. My bedroom window looked right into it with the result that I acquired an abiding hatred of Indian music! The bad thing was that the P.V.O. had been ill and more or less out of action for six weeks before his appendicitis was diagnosed, so things were in a bit of a mess. It was wonderful, however, having a proper job after so many months of wandering about and it was fun getting things straightened out. In some respects, the dairy project was a help to the province as a whole because the Governor required a monthly progress report and that enabled me to get everything I wanted from Mpwapwa including supplies for the Province itself, under the guise of the project. Already, Neil Reid had transferred a new three-ton lorry, a pick-up truck, a motor cycle, a new microscope and plenty of drugs. The Indian clerk and the African staff were OK and just needed to know that somebody cared. There was a little surgery for dogs and cats next to the office which was largely run by an African Veterinary Assistant but it was good to have the much needed opportunity to keep my hand in. The social contacts also provided a few free dinners. The pressing concern, however, was the work at the derelict air base some five miles outside Tanga.

The work in progress at the air base was organised and supervised by a relatively young Dane, probably in his thirties, who had been introduced to life in the raw in Tanganyika as an assistant manager on a sisal plantation, of which there were many in Tanga Province. He was assisted by another European whose designation and precise role I have forgotten. There were plenty of abandoned buildings around the place but the two men preferred to live under canvas in the shade of a clump of trees with their entourage of servants - male and female - and in general seemed to be a relaxed lot. Apart from the airstrip, most of the land waiting to be converted into a dairy farm was tsetse bush so the main work in progress was bush clearing, conducted by a band of about a hundred labourers armed with pangas (machetes). Teams were assigned a given area to be slashed each day. One of the conditions of service drawn up by the Dane was that each man was to bring back ten cashew nuts (*korosho*) at the end of each day when coming back to have his time sheet signed. The offerings were dropped into a sack propped against the desk to receive them. At first sight, it struck me as blatant exploitation but the labourers did not seem to resent the modest levy on the much greater quantities that they themselves took home! Anyway, I soon relaxed and began to look forward to a glass of cold beer in the cool of the evening with the blokes at the campsite and wondered how many beers one got for a sack of nuts!

Such light relief at the farm was welcome because there was East Coast fever as well as the general health of the heifers to worry about. Two more of the original herd of seventy-five were obviously ill and lymph smears confirmed that it was ECF. The dipping tank was a new one and it transpired that samples of the wash were taken into Tanga at reasonably regular intervals where the Veterinary Assistant tested them. Arsenic dips were still being used so, as described earlier, periodic testing was important. If the wash were over-strength the cattle were liable to be poisoned; if too weak, the ticks survived and the cattle were liable to die of ECF, or other tick-borne diseases. Before my arrival, the wash had been found to be grossly under-strength on several occasions and it was eventually discovered that a tap, which discharged piped water into the mixing tank, was frequently left on overnight. It then transpired that some of the locals had been sneaking into the farm after dark to draw water at the dip. That had been fixed by fitting a padlock to the tap. Nevertheless, a few more animals that had been infected before the dip was fixed died despite Bertie Lowe's order that they should not do so. Some of the blood smears that were taken from the herd at regular intervals as general routine came up positive for trypanosomes but there was an effective treatment for such cases. Fresh cases would continue to occur until the whole grazing area and the periphery had been cleared of bush, thereby depriving the tsetse fly transmitters of the shade they required for their survival.

The next problem that landed on my desk was a telegram announcing that fifty more heifers were due to arrive within the next few days.

They obviously had to be kept separate from the original herd in some kind of quarantine. By then I knew my way around Tanga and soon satisfied myself that there were no fencing materials to be had from the Public Works Department, or from any of the Indian stores. However, during my perambulations I had spotted a mass of barbed wire surrounding what looked like an abandoned air raid shelter and other military installations right in the centre of the town. As the war was over the army had apparently gone, as had the Fleet Air Arm. Since there was no time to waste, there seemed to be little point in becoming involved with bureaucracy by making a formal request to the District Commissioner, so somebody suggested I should short-circuit the process by seeking the assistance of the local jail. The Prison Officer was most helpful and promptly provided me with a gang of prisoners under the control of two armed askaris (policemen). After a little instruction they set to, detaching, disentangling and rolling up the wire. When I returned a few hours later to check the progress, the sight of the prisoners being forced at gun point to steal Government property struck me as the height of irony, especially as most of the unfortunate individuals were probably themselves serving time for very minor (unarmed!) offences. The operation reminded me of a book about East Africa by Negley Farson entitled *Behind God's Back*. In those days, one could get away with things unheard of at home!

Long before the end of my month, I was well settled in Tanga and hoped that Mpwapwa would forget about me for a few more weeks. The work was fun and at weekends there were pleasant places to go such as a magnificent, almost empty beach at Pangani only twenty miles south, where friendly Arabs could always be relied upon to take me out for a day's superb fishing. Lushoto, a hill station some sixty miles to the west, high up in the Usumbara Mountains, with its cold, moist atmosphere and forests, provided a spectacular change to the sticky heat and coconut palms of Tanga. I was living in the lap of luxury (comparatively speaking) at the hotel, all expenses paid, where there were plenty of social contacts to be made.

It was now well into November, the temperature and the humidity which had been rising steadily was becoming oppressive, so when it got too sticky there was always somebody ready to accompany one to the swimming club. It consisted merely of a hut on the edge of the nearby rocky shore, with a raft about fifty yards out in an inlet of the Indian Ocean. At the end of a sticky day it was bliss to sit on the raft dangling one's feet in the lukewarm water watching the changing colours as the golden sun dropped rapidly below the horizon to the west. At the dairy farm, a few miles to the west, more than a hundred heifers would soon be calving down, if all went well, and producing milk for Tanga. At that stage I was quite unaware that, in the opposite direction, some forty miles to the east there was a fascinating island called Pemba. I was equally unaware that, thirty-six years later I would return to what was, by then, Tanzania as a Technical Consultant for the Irish Department of Foreign Affairs to initiate a project which aimed to increase milk production for the escalating human population on the Island of Pemba. With the wisdom of hindsight, the scheme was conducted on more enlightened lines than the Tanga project involving, as it did, smallholder farmers in the ownership and management of high-yielding local Zebu/Jersey cross-bred cows. As will be detailed more fully later, the smallholder system proved to be infinitely more rewarding socially and, in the long term, more cost effective and sustainable under what was by then Tanzanian conditions than large Government owned enterprises.

But in November 1946 there were signs that my cushy life at Tanga had not long to go. Carl Anderson, had been relieved at Lake Province and arrived to take over the dairy farm. Hugh Newlands, who was out of hospital and convalescing at Lushoto, had been looking so well on my last visit that I could not resist telling him that it was now appallingly hot in Tanga; I urged him to take his time! My desire to linger longer in Tanga was intensified one night as I breezed into the hotel dining room and was brought up short by the sight of a large party which included four beautiful girls who I soon learnt were aged sixteen to twenty-five. The sudden appearance of a whole family of girls in Tanga was enough to make me pause momentarily, straighten my tie and inspect my nails before wending my way to my own table. As I sat down, one of the girls, a pretty redhead waved across the room and gave me a cheery smile. Good grief! It was Ruth, the girl I had lost on the train between Moshi and Tanga, a month ago! In due course, the girls and two of the older folk, obviously Mother and Father, rose from the table and as they made for the door Ruth joined me, chatted for a while and then invited me to have coffee with the family. Introductions all round: 'Rob, this is Mum, Dad, Pearl, Audrey, Elizabeth'. Two blondes, a brunette, a redhead and cordial, well-disposed parents all together in Tanga - unbelievable. Everything went so well that I was invited to go along with them to the cinema. Over a nightcap, the father and I seemed to get on well; he told me that he owned a power station at Korogwe that provided electricity for Tanga and the numerous sisal estates in the area. He finished up by inviting me to spend a weekend with them all on my next visit to Lushoto. This was great! The anticlimax came a few days later in the form of a telegram that instructed me to hand over to Carl Anderson, to proceed forthwith by road to Mpwapwa (over 300 miles away) for a conference which was to be attended by all the vets in the country. I was to bring my loads with me; that was the end of Tanga. Fate had ordained that my promising friendship with Ruth was to end, as two ships that had passed (twice!) in the night, never to meet again!

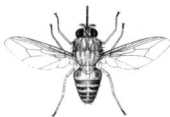

CHAPTER TWENTY

Back to Mpwapwa

Changes at Mpwapwa. Case work in the laboratory. Continued world shortage of vegetable oils results in the conception of the ill-fated 'groundnut scheme' which would eventually cost British taxpayers millions of pounds. An account of the initiation and subsequent failure of the scheme.

Arriving back at Mpwapwa was like coming home, not just to familiar surroundings but also to people who were more like family than friends. That feeling heightened when I arrived at CJ's house where I was to stay during the conference. Since our last meeting he had managed to secure an outward passage from the Isle of Man for his fiancée. He was now a happily married man and while Mona welcomed me with open arms CJ stood to one side, smiling smugly. The former bachelor's abode had been softened and oozed domesticity.

The conference was a great success having brought together from far and wide all of the sixteen vets, other than Hugh Newlands, who were by then in the country. After the day's work the social life, augmented by accompanying wives, went on into the small hours and created a great buzz in the confines of Kikombo. It was a very different Mpwapwa.

During the conference the Director told me that although I was now entitled to home leave it was unlikely to be granted for another year. It was some compensation, however, to learn that my perambulations were over for the moment and that I would almost certainly remain at Mpwapwa for the rest of my tour. After the departure of the visitors, Jack Wilde filled me in on the details. I was to join him at the laboratory where I would be in charge of the material coming from the field for laboratory diagnosis, and responsible for the health of the livestock on the station. I would also assist Jack with his research on rinderpest and trypanosomiasis but would be free to do some research of my own on conditions affecting the Mpwapwa livestock. There were plans to establish a post of Veterinary Education Officer to resume the training of African Veterinary Assistants, so I was asked to prepare the courses if time permitted. Jack was even more enthusiastic after his home leave which had been extended for special studies than he had been the previous year and had exciting plans for the development of the laboratory. His staff had already been increased by the arrival of a young chemist and a laboratory technician from England. His enthusiasm was infectious and I was delighted at the prospect of settling down under his guidance. I was so impressed by his many talents and accomplishments; he had an ability to put his hand to anything from photography, to oil painting, golf, repairing boilers, and pulling teeth for the labourers. He had a sense of fun and zest for life; all this made the next seven months a turning point in my life. It was also the beginning of a friendship with him and his wife Kathleen that induced me to join them five years later in Nigeria where, in due course, they first met my young bride, Joyce. Kathleen is loved by us both to this day.

I had the good fortune to be allocated a fine house almost next door to the laboratory and lost no time in unpacking my household gear, which had been stored at Mpwapwa since my departure from Tabora almost six months previously. It was a relief to settle down amongst the old treasures after my nomadic existence in bush. In contrast, Selemani was not as pleased as me to be back in Mpwapwa. During his time at Tanga he had become homesick for the Coast and for some time had been much quieter than usual. Eventually, with his characteristic hunching of the shoulders and swaying from the hips with eyes to the ground he explained that he wanted to go home. It was rather sad for the two of us but not particularly so for Jackson who, in due course, offered to double up as cook cum house servant with the assistance of a garden boy. The new arrangement soon proved to be a success as Jackson applied himself to the abundance of good things which had, by then, become available from the *dukas* in Mpwapwa village. He proved to be an excellent cook and general factotum. It was just as well, because the social life had changed. Standards had risen and it was time to throw a few sundowners and dinner parties in return for the generous hospitality I had been receiving. The social changes were to some extent due to the increase in the population of expatriates, both at the lab and at Headquarters, but even more so to the influx of wives who had eventually managed to get passages back to Tanganyika after extended periods at home. There was even a 'Lady Administrative Assistant' at Headquarters. During my first year there were only three expatriate wives in the Kikombo valley and they had fitted comfortably into what was essentially a rather monastic community made up of bachelors and grass widowers who were held together by their mutual interest in the work. It was no longer the man's world that it had been during my first year. There was more company at the tennis court and swimming pool, couples were occasionally seen on the little golf course and the sundowners that followed these and other afternoon activities were less likely, in the presence of the ladies, to degenerate into the wilder drinking bouts that had been so effective in easing tensions that had periodically built up in the former male-dominated society.

The Director's wife was now back after prolonged leave at home and it was clear that the 'Big House' and, indeed the Director himself, were very much under new management. This was very evident on Christmas night when all of the twenty-two Europeans on the station sat down to dinner at the Big House. The ladies, dressed in evening gowns, and the men, in white dinner jackets and black ties, were served the traditional turkey, ham, and Christmas pudding by servants in spotlessly white *kanzus* set off with colourful cummerbunds. After dinner the ladies retired to the sitting room while the men sat over their coffee and South African brandy before all coming together again for charades and other party games. The following night there was a buffet supper for all down at the headmaster's house just beyond the village of Mpwapwa outside the veterinary enclave. The pattern had been set - it was black ties again! As we looked out from the veranda across the vast, moonlit plains of Gogoland and listened to the beat of drums from the nearby village the intrusion of the new-found formality seemed, to some of us, decidedly out of place.

It was good to be back to hands-on veterinary work at the lab, after the administrative chore of running Western Province and, worse still, killing time in bush waiting for the next telegram from Mpwapwa. Now that I had more time at my disposal I was particularly pleased to have responsibility for the clinical work involving the two thousand or so head of cattle, sheep, goats and pigs, plus the zoo animals and the poultry. It was more like the work of a general practitioner at home, with the added advantage of having the laboratory facilities with which to investigate the clinical problems in greater depth with a view to devising preventive measures. In retrospect, it is interesting to contemplate the paucity of diagnostic procedures, drugs and vaccines that were available in those days to the veterinarian for the treatment and control of the many important diseases then prevalent not only in Tanganyika but also throughout the rest of the world. It is also interesting to compare the situation then with the extraordinary advances that were subsequently made during the second half of the century. The paucity of effective drugs in those days is well illustrated by the high, uncontrollable prevalence of two particular parasitic infestations of sheep and goats at Mpwapwa at that time, namely the sheep nasal fly, *Oestrus ovis*, and the blood-sucking worm *Haemonchus contortus*.

Oestrus ovis is a robust fly, about 1 cm long and, having only rudimentary mouth parts, it does not feed so it is entirely parasitic on sheep during its larval stages. These occur in the nasal passages of their host. Unlike its close cousin the warble fly, which used to cause great distress to cattle and the destruction of hides in temperate climes, it does not lay eggs; instead, it hovers in the vicinity of the sheep's muzzle and, at the first opportunity, squirts a jet of liquid containing some twenty larvae at a time on to the nostrils of the host. At this stage, the larvae are only about 1 mm long. It is fascinating to contemplate how the attraction of the fly to the precise vicinity of the nostrils and, in particular, the technique for the delivery of the tiny larvae evolved. Presumably, it did so during the course of countless generations long before the fly was first described by Linnaeus in 1761. Even at that early date the fly was well ahead of today's military aircraft that now use a rather similar technique for the delivery of their air-to-ground missiles. The hovering of the fly in the vicinity of the muzzle causes great distress to the sheep who close ranks tightly, stamp their feet, and do their best to squeeze their heads deep into the fleece of their companions. First stage larvae that have been successfully delivered onto the nostrils migrate into the nasal passages, some going as far as the nasal sinuses. While in the nasal passages they attach themselves by means of oral hooks to the mucous membrane on which they are nourished and eventually grow, after a series of moult, to a robust length of some 3 cm. The presence of the larvae in the nasal passages produces a copious discharge of mucous. As a result, practically all of the sheep at Mpwapwa, and indeed many of the goats, showed a rather nauseating discharge of slimy exudate from the nose at almost any given time of the year. Needless to say, the attention of the fly as well as the presence of the larvae affected the general welfare and productivity of the sheep and goats. On completion of the larval development the mature larvae either crawl or are sneezed out of the nasal passage and fall to the ground where they pupate. In duc course, an adult fly emerges which is presumably genetically determined to locate a sheep and to squirt a new generation of larvae into the nostrils, thereby completing the remarkable lifecycle.

There was no effective treatment for the alleviation of this distressing condition until the chlorinated hydrocarbon hexachlorethane became available as an insecticide in the late forties. Unfortunately, the delivery of the drug involved holding each sheep on its back while a suspension of the drug in oil was instilled into the nostrils. Such a technique was not practicable where large numbers of animals were involved. However, systemic insecticides subsequently became available which destroy practically all the larvae in the nasal passages when appropriate preparations are administered either by mouth, or simply poured on to the skin from where the insecticide is carried to the larvae in the deepest recesses of the nasal chambers. The treatment of the entire sheep and goat populations on two or three occasions during the course of a single year would probably eradicate the fly from isolated flocks and herds such as those at Mpwapwa. Unfortunately, for many years past the main difficulty in undertaking programmes of this kind in tropical Africa against *Oestrus ovis* and other parasites has been the shortage of funds for the purchase of the many excellent drugs now on the market.

A much more serious threat to the health and, indeed, the survival of the sheep and goats at Mpwapwa was parasitic gastro-enteritis caused by the acquisition of a variety of tiny parasitic worms from the pastures during the rains. The most lethal of these was *Haemonchus contortus,* which lived in the abomasum, that is, the fourth stomach of cattle, sheep and goats. It could be easily recognised lying there on the inner surface of the stomach by its bright red colour, indicating the presence of blood in its intestine. In heavily infested lambs and kids the mortality rate was high and although older animals were rather more resistant continuous exposure to infection seriously affected their productivity. The treatment at Mpwapwa in those days involved the drenching of all of the sheep and goats with a weak solution of copper sulphate at intervals of two weeks during the wet season. It was a time-consuming procedure that, even at such short intervals, left much to be desired in terms of effectiveness. Nowadays, with the acquisition of greatly increased knowledge of the biology of the parasite coupled with the advent of modern, highly efficient drugs, the problem can be effectively controlled by two or three treatments during the year, administered at judiciously chosen intervals.

While some changes had taken place at Mpwapwa during 1946 they were soon to pale into utter insignificance when compared with what was being planned in London, and elsewhere, for the Mpwapwa District. The very name Mpwapwa, though not the veterinary enclave, was to become world famous. Those who experienced the food rationing in Great Britain during the Second World War will recall that the greatest deprivation was the shortage of butter and other edible oils. Harassed British housewives had looked forward to the end of the war when unlimited supplies of New Zealand butter would once again appear in the shops. No doubt, they also assumed that vegetable oils would soon flow unhindered from all parts of the world to Unilever's Port Sunlight at Liverpool for the manufacture of much needed margarine, soap and many other scarce commodities. This did not happen; instead rationing continued for several years and on occasions the butter quota was actually cut. The reason for this was that, despite the carnage that had taken place in the theatres of war, the population of the world had actually continued to rise steadily during the period 1938 to 1945. By the end of the war it was estimated that there were globally more than one hundred and twenty million extra mouths to feed. The shortage of vegetable oils was also exacerbated by the destruction of oil palm and coconut plantations during the hostilities in the Far East.

The shortage was of great concern to the British Government for obvious reasons, but also to Unilever whose vast commercial enterprise was so dependent on adequate supplies of animal fats and vegetable oils. In Africa and the Far East, Unilever had extensive plantations of their own for the production of palm oil and coconut oil and also purchased palm-kernel nuts, copra, oil-rich groundnuts, rape seed, cotton seed, sunflower seed, and linseed throughout the world. Because of the urgency of the problem there was no point in considering extending the plantations of oil or coconut palms because of their slow generation time; instead, attention would have to be given to an annual crop such as the groundnut. The thought of groundnuts turned attention to parts of Africa where there was no shortage of uninhabited land, much of which was probably suitable for groundnuts. Most of Unilever's extensive business in Africa was conducted by one of its subsidiaries, the United Africa Company (UAC) which, among many other activities, purchased huge quantities of groundnuts from smallholders in Northern Nigeria. Great pyramids of sacks filled with these nuts, waiting for transport by rail to Lagos, were an architectural feature of Kano during the dry season.

At the beginning of 1946, the Chief Executive of UAC went to Tanzania and was greatly impressed by the vast expanses of uninhabited bush that he saw during his tour around the country. During discussions with the Department of Agriculture it was suggested that UAC might consider growing 20,000 acres of groundnuts on a rotational basis with other appropriate crops involving a total of 100,000 acres. A plantation approach that would, of necessity, be entirely dependent on mechanisation rather than a multiplicity of smallholder enterprises was envisaged. This was big thinking for Tanganyika yet it transpired to be only a fraction of what was eventually undertaken. Back in London, after further consultations, the Chief Executive of UAC submitted an ambitious scheme to the Minister of Food involving the clearance of 2,555,000 acres for the cultivation of groundnuts. A fundamental concept was that an economic return from such a large-scale undertaking could be achieved only by the clearance of bush and the subsequent cultivation and harvesting of the crop by mechanical means. Shortly thereafter, the proposed scheme was accepted in principle by the Government and a three-man delegation headed by a distinguished authority on tropical agriculture, who had spent the early part of his career in the Colonial Agricultural Service in Tanganyika, was appointed to investigate the feasibility of the scheme.

The delegation arrived in East Africa in June 1946 and spent approximately two months searching for suitable sites mainly in Tanganyika but also in Kenya and Northern Rhodesia. In Tanganyika it initially favoured an area of 1,650,000 acres in Southern Province and another 300,000 acres near Tabora in Western Province. However, while they were still in the country, they were contacted by my old friend Bwana Bain, whose herd of pigs at Mlali had given me so much anguish during my first year at the laboratory. He invited the delegation to visit him and inspect the country at the back of the mountains some twelve miles north of Mpwapwa, as the crow flies.

As things turned out it might have saved the British taxpayer millions of pounds during the next two or three years if he had not intervened and the delegation had contented itself with a pilot scheme further up the railway line at Tabora. Instead, the party flew from Dar es Salaam and presumably landed on the airstrip at the Veterinary Department's Lower Farm near Mpwapwa village. They would have been met there by Bwana Bain and driven in his battered box-bodied car from Mpwapwa along the dusty, dry-season road to Matamonda, then across the mountains to Mlali and on a little further to his house perched on the hillside. As they emerged from the car and, no doubt, turned around to see where they had come from, they must have been greatly impressed by the vast expanse of dead-flat thorn bush, interspersed with a few hills and patches of grassland that lay stretching to the west and the north as far as the eye could see. That night, apart from a few flickering lights at the nearby village of Mlali, there would have been no other lights to be seen; beyond Mlali the vast area was practically uninhabited and, as things turned out, was theirs for the asking.

With characteristic enthusiasm Bwana Bain took them careering round the country, more often than not having to hack roads into the almost impenetrable bush to ascertain whether the soil was of the type required for groundnuts. Near the tiny village of Kongwa, at the other side of the Kiborani Mountains from Mpwapwa and some twenty-five miles west of Mlali, the visitors saw some plots of groundnuts and subsequent checks indicated that the yield was very satisfactory. Sadly, they did not realise that the rainfall just to the north where the whole Kongwa enterprise was to be undertaken was the lowest in Tanganyika and, worse still, it was largely unpredictable. However, the delegation was so impressed by the general area that they added another 450,000 acres to their list of 1,650,000 and 300,000 acres that they had decided should be developed in Southern Province and Western Province, respectively. After their return to the U.K in September 1946 they recommended that the scheme should be developed in units of 30,000. Eighty units would be established in Tanganyika of which fifteen units (450,000 acres) would be at Kongwa, seventeen in Northern Rhodesia and ten in Kenya. The capital cost of the whole scheme, to be spread over six years, was estimated to be some £24,000,000, a staggering amount in those days. When this sum is converted into today's value its expenditure over such a short period gives a good measure of the magnitude of the undertaking and the urgency with which it was approached.

The delegation's report seems to have been accepted with incredible, almost feverish, enthusiasm by practically all concerned, including the British Government. Almost immediately, Unilever began searching all over the world for second-hand bulldozers and heavy tractors because there was no hope of purchasing such a large quantity of new equipment in time. Just before Christmas, presumably while the Director's wife and the other good ladies at Mpwapwa were planning to raise the ante over Christmas and placing their orders for festive hams with Bwana Bain, a decision was announced in London which, amongst many other things, would place impossible demands on the Mlali pigs for the production of the next year's hams. To be precise, the decision was that the first phase of the whole Groundnut Scheme would begin on the 450,000 acres at the back of the mountains behind Mpwapwa!

The decision was received with considerable scepticism by those at Mpwapwa and others who knew the area well. They were dumfounded that such a vast and perilous undertaking, based largely on aspirations rather than on facts acquired from appropriate feasibility studies, was about to be launched on their very doorstep. The early planners were warned that the single-line, narrow-gauge Central Railway from Dar-es-Salaam would be quite incapable of coping with the huge volume of heavy equipment, cement, fuel and all manner of other materials that would have to be transported to Kongwa in a short space of time. It was also explained that during the rains stretches of the line through the hilly country between Kilosa and Gulwe were regularly washed away and, as there was no road to the coast, Mpwapwa was frequently cut off for days on end. Their attention was also drawn to difficulties the Veterinary Department had always encountered in employing the local Wagogo people. It had to be expected that those we regarded as permanent labourers, or even semi-skilled staff, could not be relied upon to turn up consistently. The Laboratory work took second place to that of their own *shambas* and at other times some just stayed at home when the fancy took them. The excuse for such absence was usually '*homo*, Bwana' (fever). In order to keep labour-intensive work such as bush clearing going, we were obliged to recruit with difficulty gangs of labourers on six month contracts from the Wabena tribe in Southern Highlands. These warnings to the 'groundnutters' invariably evoked even greater enthusiasm. The need for oils was such that all these difficulties would just have to be overcome; the fundamental problem was that so many of the planners, and those being recruited, had just been directly or indirectly involved in a war in which great feats had been achieved without any consideration of the cost of the materials and the human effort involved. They would soon find that a commercial operation would prove to be a different matter.

Early in February 1947, some two months after I had returned to Mpwapwa, an advance party of key men arrived in the middle of the night at Gulwe station. Next morning they were driven through the village of Mpwapwa along the road to Mlali that leads past Matamonda to the back of the mountains. There they joined a white hunter who had set up a camp of sorts beside a pleasant little stream at a spot called Sagara, some ten miles to the west of Mlali. It was here, at the back-of-beyond, that the newcomers began to face the practical realities of transforming the vast plain on which they now stood into a farm of 450,000 acres. Before long, they moved their tents twelve miles further west to the tiny village of Kongwa at the other end of the mountains which was to become the permanent headquarters of the scheme. Almost immediately, work started at Msagali, ten miles to the west of Gulwe Station, on a branch line to join Kongwa to the Central Railway line. From that point on successive waves of new recruits began to arrive at Dar es Salaam to staff the offices and depots there and begin the actual operations at Kongwa. For the best part of a year, all the staff at Kongwa from the highest to the lowest lived under canvas in extremely difficult conditions. Eventually permanent and semi-permanent housing was erected for expatriate and African staff including indigenous labour that was recruited and drawn in from many parts of Tanganyika. In the fullness of time the tiny village of Kongwa grew into a sizeable town complete with an excellent hospital and other social amenities, as well as workshops and stores for the business in hand.

The initial target for the general area of Kongwa was the clearing and planting of 150,000 acres (thirty units) of bush during 1947. For this area alone, 200 bulldozers would be required. The biggest stocks available turned out to be in the Philippines where large numbers had been left behind by American forces. Those that were purchased were transported across the Indian Ocean but sadly many of these proved to have seen better times and caused much frustration in the early days before workshops and stocks of much needed spares had been established. On the first attempt to get them up to Msagali by rail the prognostications of the Mpwapwa sceptics about the inadequacy of the Central Railway were proved right; the blades of the bulldozers were too wide for some of the cuttings. The latter had to be widened by means of the old-reliable *pangas* and *jembes* (slashers and hoes). Concurrently, supplies of all kinds such as trucks, tents, electric generators, workshop machinery and spare parts, as well as all sorts of bizarre 'bargains' which subsequently proved useless were being purchased from war-disposal centres in the Middle East, Europe and even West Africa. Because of the congestion in the harbour at Dar es Salaam some of these supplies had to be brought overland along hazardous dirt-roads all the way from Nairobi in ex-Army lorries which had seen service in the Western Desert - not an easy task during the rains.

The bush-clearance began by cutting parallel tracks, the width of the bulldozer, a mile apart into the bush. Further parallel tracks were then cut at right angles to these, also a mile apart, thus producing a chequerboard composed of square mile sections. The bulldozers then set to, attempting to clear the bush section by section. The next problem was to dispose of the thick cover of felled bush, so contour lines were pegged out at appropriate intervals and the bush was pushed by the bulldozers to form windrows along the contour lines. Apart from disposing of the bush, this device was also intended to prevent soil erosion during the rains and to minimise wind erosion in the long dry season. (See illusts.) But this proved to be only a preliminary step in preparing a seed-bed; the thorn bush that had probably been there untouched by human-hand for centuries, if ever, had put a tangled network of tough roots deep into the soil. Conventional rooters proved incapable of tearing up or even cutting the interlacing mass and after much trial and error a new tool designed specifically for the job had to be manufactured in England. In the meantime, clearance of the bush-cover continued but even this was impeded by the continuous breakdown of the second-hand bulldozers, the inadequacy of the workshops and the almost complete absence of spares. As a consequence, by the end of June 1947, when I left Mpwapwa on home leave, only 1,027 acres had been cleared though. In August, the belated arrival of more tractors brought the intended complement up to 200 and by the end of October 12,000 acres had been cleared. However, by the time planting was to begin during the short rains over Christmas three quarters of the tractors were out of action and only 7,500 acres had been cleared of roots, thereby providing a seedbed just about acceptable for planting. All sorts of logistical difficulties were encountered in acquiring and modifying machinery for mechanical planting in the conditions encountered at Kongwa. Nevertheless, although the planting of the 7,500 acres fell far short of the 150,000 target, thanks to the heroic efforts of those involved who worked during the day and night under appallingly difficult conditions, a great expanse of groundnuts was up and ready for harvesting four months later, albeit at enormous expense.

By then, I was far away from Mpwapwa and destined not to return to the Mlali/Kongwa area until 1992. In retrospect, it is unfortunate that the first year's operations were not regarded as a pilot exercise on the basis of which realistic plans might have been drawn up. Instead, the programme was allowed to proceed by a system of trial and error in the hope of achieving what proved to be utterly hopeless aspirations. It seems, however, that the momentum could not be stopped. By 1949, there was a town, large by Tanganyikan standards, stuck out in the blue at Kongwa complete with an excellent hospital, a large shop selling consumer goods to a multi-racial society, cinemas and social clubs. The fundamental scheme, the growing of groundnuts, was tinkered with by such devices as diversification into sunflowers and eventually cattle ranching. A severe drought during 1949, which was a periodic feature of the climate of the

Ugogo plains, devastated the first sunflower crop and reduced the yield of groundnuts. Eventually it was accepted that growing groundnuts on such a massive scale at Kongwa was not an economic proposition and it seems that the scheme petered out during the fifties. The projects in the Southern Highlands and in Western Province also ran into extreme difficulties and the extension of the scheme to Kenya and Zambia never took place.

★

When I returned to the Kogwa area in 1992, there was nothing to be seen of the groundnut plantations, or indeed of the town itself. As shown in the illustration, there had been no regeneration of the original dense cover of thorn bush; such grass as there was had been eaten down to the roots exposing the brown soil to wind erosion. The village of Mlali and the surrounding country had by then become more heavily populated by humans, cattle, sheep and goats, and soil erosion, as shown by the extensive rivers of sand, had reached an advanced state. There were far too many cattle around and the shortage of grass had driven many of them into the tsetse bush on the hills to the south. As a result cases of trypanosomiasis were prevalent. One of the most disappointing features of my visit was my failure to trace even a foundation of Bwana Bain's house and factory on the side of the mountain overlooking the village. It was sad indeed to find that Bwana Bain and his little family, whose enthusiasm had brought so much life and prosperity to the village of Mlali before the Groundnut Scheme had even been dreamt of, had disappeared without trace as had the very pigs themselves.

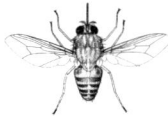

CHAPTER TWENTY-ONE

From Mpwapwa to the Bright Lights of Piccadilly

Final months of work at Mpwapwa. Research into tuberculosis in cattle. An illness and four weeks in hospital in Dar es Salaam. Reflections on the tour of service and whether it might be the last. The journey home - a quick four days by air, compared to the three month outward voyage. Reflections on the impact of war and peacetime on relationships, and on the people and city of London. Back home to family and a new job.

While great things were happening at Kongwa in 1947 the work at Mpwapwa continued at a less frenetic pace, at least as far as I was concerned. My responsibilities for the health of the stock left me plenty of time to assist Jack with his own research on trypanosomiasis and East Coast fever and also to choose a research topic for myself. During 1946 there had been a generalised case of tuberculosis in one of the lab cattle and tuberculin testing had revealed fifteen reactors in the dairy herd. This in itself was a serious business because although most of the households that bought milk at the dairy boiled the milk as a routine precaution against bacterial infections, most of the labourers probably did not do so. A much bigger problem vis-à-vis bovine tuberculosis existed in the Southern Highlands and Bukoba where the incidence of the disease was high and it was intended to address the problem as soon as staff levels improved. In the meantime, the presence of infections at Mpwapwa provided an opportunity to do some work on diagnostic techniques.

The testing procedure for tuberculosis used in Great Britain and Ireland in those days involved clipping the hair from a small patch on the side of the neck, measuring a fold of the skin on the bare area and then injecting a drop of tuberculin - an extract of the bacterium *Mycobacterium tuberculosis* - into the thickness of the skin at that precise point. The site was examined after an appropriate interval and in some cases injected again, but in all instances the criterion on which one based a positive diagnosis was the development of a characteristic, diffuse thickening at the site of injection. While I was contemplating various permutations of the test I learnt that the Director of the Veterinary Laboratory of the Ministry of Agriculture at Stormont, Northern Ireland was, at that particular time, engaged on a critical study of tuberculin testing. At one stage in the investigations he had injected the tuberculin intradermally into a fold of skin at the base of the tail known as the caudal fold. This seemed the obvious site for use on a mass scale in Tanganyika because cattle were seldom housed; they were simply grazed in herds by day under the supervision of a herd boy and spent the night in fenced enclosures, *boma*s. During inoculation campaigns cattle were simply driven into rather crude, narrow crushes in which they instinctively lowered their heads as close to the ground as possible. Tuberculin testing on a mass scale would have been impossible in these circumstances, so it was decided to compare the reliability of the caudal fold test with that of the conventional procedure which used the skin on the side of the neck.

Here it should be explained that there are three morphologically indistinguishable types of *M. tuberculosis*; namely the bovine type, the human and the avian. The bovine type is by far the most common type found in cattle and in those days, before pasteurisation of milk was practised to any extent, its incidence in man was also high. For example, in 1932 it was estimated that infection of humans with the bovine type was responsible for 5.2 per cent of the total deaths from tuberculosis in man in England and Wales. Lesions caused by the bovine type in man are much more common in the lymphatic system than elsewhere in the body. Indeed, as a student in Dublin, I remember being impressed by the remarkable number of people one passed in the streets who had a scar on the side of the neck marking the point from which tuberculous cervical lymph nodes had been excised. Most, if not all, of these infections had resulted from the drinking of cow's milk, rather than by inhalation, so the scarred necks reflected graphically the distressingly high prevalence of mammary tuberculosis in the dairy herds throughout the country. The bovine type infection in man was not, however, confined to the lymphatic system; a proportion of the cases of tuberculosis of the bone and joints was bovine in origin and one of the most lethal and tragic manifestations of the infection was meningitis in infants.

The human type has a much narrower range of hosts and actual lesions are only occasionally found in cattle, though its entry into the tissues of the animal is capable of sensitising the skin, which is then likely to react positively to bovine tuberculin. The avian type rarely produces detectable lesions in cattle but, here again, the mere entry of the tubercles into the body may sensitise the skin.

The actual tuberculin test using either the caudal fold site or the side of the neck was, of course, a simple undertaking that was got under way without difficulty, but evaluation of the results was a different story. The animals that showed a positive reaction were slaughtered one by one and all of the major lymph nodes, particularly those in the chest and abdominal cavities, as well as visceral organs such as the lung, liver, spleen, kidneys, ovaries, uterus and mammary gland were examined for the presence of the characteristic tuberculous lesions, as were the pericardium and the linings of the thoracic and peritoneal cavities. The major lymph nodes were then excised and sliced into thin slivers and examined for minute tuberculous nodules. Smears were taken on glass slides from any suspicious spots for microscopic examination. The smears were then stained by a specific technique which, under the microscope, showed the tubercule bacilli's characteristic morphology in red, while other morphologically similar bacteria were stained blue.

Unfortunately, it proved impossible to find the tubercule bacillus in the majority of those that had reacted positively to the tuberculin test, irrespective of whether the injection had been made into the skin of the caudal fold or the neck. A possible explanation was that the high prevalence of false positive reactions had resulted from the mere exposure of the cattle to the avian type or, much less likely, to the human type of *Mycobacterium tuberculosis*, or even to other species of the genus. Therefore, it was important at this stage to identify the actual type of *M. tuberculosis* recovered from a reactor in which tuberculous abscesses or even tiny, suspicious lesions had been found. There were two ways of doing this.

One involved artificial infection of laboratory animals, namely rabbits, guinea-pigs and chickens, with suspect material and comparing the nature and duration of the reactions in the different species over a period of up to three months. The other method was based on determining the ability of any of the isolated organisms to grow on different culture media and studying the rate of growth and other characteristics of any of the growths obtained. In view of the cruelty involved in the first method, there was no difficulty in opting for the second method though, as things turned out, it proved immensely frustrating because of my inadequate knowledge of practical bacteriology.

During the practical classes at the Veterinary College we had been given ample opportunity to study bacteria under the microscope but we were only shown cultures of some of the more easily grown species; the preparation of culture media and the growth of the organisms was done by a technician in a side-lab. Consequently, at Mpwapwa I had to take down a big tome and delve into the wonderful world of practical bacteriology. The preferred medium on which to grow T.B. was Dorset Egg Medium. Being so far from England, my initial reaction was, 'Oh no! Will Mpwapwa eggs be O.K.?' Then I noticed that a Mr Kauffman, a Mr Schawbacker and many others were all famous for having devised their own particular egg medium; Messers Petrof and Malkani had included a generous quantity of beef broth and added a dash of glycerine. A Mr Petragani must have been at it longer because he had eventually added milk, slices of potatoes, a little glycerine and finally a few drops of malachite green to the eggs; his lab assistant was probably Irish-American! So many had been at it that it seemed that the *in vitro* cultivation of *M. tuberculosis*, and presumably many other bacteria, had evolved by trial and error rather than from a biochemical study of their nutritional requirements. When one turned to the section on the preparation of the actual media it seemed to have been written by Mrs Beaton; literally 'take a dozen eggs'! The procedure was complicated by the fact that the final concoction could not be sterilised simply by putting it in the autoclave; the eggs would have been scrambled. Instead, the eggshells had to be sterilised, so that the egg white and yolks could be removed aseptically. The mixing of the eggs with the other ingredients and the transfer of the whole concoction into the final glass containers also had to be done aseptically, as if it were a surgical operation. In addition, everything used – instruments, other ingredients, glassware, even hands and towels – had to be sterilised during the various procedures until the culture medium was 'seeded' (inoculated) with the tuberculous material, which had also been processed to destroy any extraneous contaminants. There were many pitfalls and false starts for the beginner before the seeded cultures were safely in the incubator. Unfortunately, before I reached that stage in what was to be an intriguing though, at times, a frustrating investigation the programme was interrupted by an even more frustrating four weeks in Dar es Salaam Hospital.

I had gradually become aware of a pain in my chest which eventually persuaded me to consult Dr Dikshit, the Assistant Surgeon in Mpwapwa. On sounding my chest he made the dramatic diagnosis of pericarditis and announced that I would have to be referred to Dar es Salaam without delay. Jack immediately gave me sick leave whereupon the news spread in the small community and within two days I was seen off by train from Gulwe to Dar by kind friends who seemed to be more convinced about the diagnosis and more concerned than I was. The four weeks in the hospital, located in a sylvan setting close to the beach, turned out to be a rather enjoyable, relaxing time with pleasant company in a spacious, high-vaulted ward cooled by the sea breezes. After the first X-ray I was relieved when the doctor told me that there was no sign of percarditis. Then he spoilt it by adding that there was a slight shadow on the surface of the lung and because of the work I had been doing it had to be investigated. From that point on I was more or less confined to bed for the rest of the month while I was monitored by regular blood tests and further X-rays. In due course, with the chest pain a thing of the past, the tedium of confinement was relieved by the company of two entertaining companions in the neighbouring beds and even more so by the visits of two cheery nurses who, despite their relative youth, had the official Colonial Service title of Nursing Sister. They were much in demand in the social round of Dar and seldom failed, before leaving to enjoy their nightlife, to give us a good laugh by strutting and pirouetting provokingly along the highly polished floor in front of us for critical appraisal of their various ensembles. A sort of 'How am I doing boys?' Towards the end of my stay I made, or rather renewed, another social contact. One day I happened to look down from the ward, which was located on the first floor, and saw a familiar figure striding past in a long white *kanzu* with a white cap precariously balanced on the forehead. I was so taken aback that I blurted out "*Namna* so-an-so *gani*, Selemani", to which I received an appropriate reply! Poor Selemani had obtained a fairly menial job in the hospital and was not allowed to visit the wards. However, we did manage to meet again before I left.

Entertaining though the sojourn was, it was a great relief to be given a clean bill of health after the last X-ray at the end of the month. Back at Mpwapwa, I had a wonderful reception from Jackson who I found actually slashing firewood for the makeshift boiler for the bath, an unusual thing for a house servant to do. He explained that the garden boy had run away after my departure and had probably joined the Groundnut Scheme for the big money, as many other house servants were doing. Labour was at a premium. Despite this, the house was in spanking order and my good friends, the Buckleys and others, had provided Jackson with the necessary perishables for the fridge and other groceries to get me going. Jack was away at a conference in Nairobi and as the new Laboratory Technician, who had been left in charge, had gone down with a cracking go of malaria I was very happy to feel well rested and badly needed at the lab again. The most exciting thing, however, was that Bertie Lowe had jumped the gun while I was in hospital by recommending me for home leave. The papers were already in Dar and I was likely to get a passage in May or June, then only three or four months away.

It was wonderful being able to dash off a letter telling the family that I would be home soon, hopefully in time for my sister's wedding. My sea-faring brother-in-law to-be, Tommy, was also due home in the spring and was determined to marry Anna while on leave, whether or not the doctor allowed her out of bed for the occasion. My brother, having been demobbed from the Navy, was at home studying for his Fellowship in surgery. On top of that, he was kept busy during the terrible freeze-up of 1947 trying to keep everybody in the family from freezing. Coal was still practically unobtainable in Ireland, coal gas was turned on by the Gas Company only for a short period before meal times, the heaps of turf stored outdoors in the Phoenix Park were sodden; so between lectures my brother was spending much of his time hunting for scrap timber, even old furniture, to dry out the wet turf. A letter from my mother told me that she and my father were going to brave the slow train to Belfast merely for the relief of sitting at a friend's coal fire for a weekend! It was a terrible time for them all. Consequently, the end of the winter could not come quickly enough for them and, now, the prospect of a wedding and my homecoming was the light at the end of the tunnel.

Despite the waiting, the interim period at Mpwapwa was quietly enjoyable. About this time a bright young graduate, Renault Beakbane, arrived to take up a position in chemistry but he was very versatile and game for anything so before long he was working more or less as a research assistant for Jack. With the increase in staff, housing accommodation was becoming scarce so I was asked if I would share my house with him. I readily did so and enjoyed his cheery company until the end of my tour. My memories of the time are of pleasantly unhurried days at the lab with some satisfying progress, punctuated with much frustration in my efforts to grow the wretched TB on various media. I remember the greenness of our surroundings following the onset of the rains that added to the pleasure of little safaris either for business or leisure. In the evenings the monotony of solo dinners was broken by frequent gatherings of bachelors at short notice in the houses of the recently married Wildes and the Buckleys for Lancashire hot-pot, Cornish pasties and other home-cooked fare, followed by a game of darts, table skittles or a few hands of cards, all accompanied by mugs of beer, merriment and happy banter. The almost suburban atmosphere, so absent during my first year at Mpwapwa, was a pleasant foretaste of what lay ahead on the forthcoming home leave. Sometimes, as one emerged into the dark emptiness of Africa, leaving the chatter and laughter behind, and made one's way home by the light of a lantern, surrounded by the chirping of the cicadas, one was struck by the incongruity of it all – a tiny oasis of European domesticity plonked down amidst such isolation.

Our isolation was brought home to us while returning from a memorable weekend safari that Jack and Kathleen Wilde, Ray Rainer and I made to an idyllic site near Mlali. Ray, a middle-aged bachelor, was the office manager at Headquarters and as such was very much the office type with little experience of the wide, open spaces. The excuse for the trip was to visit Renault Beakbane who was busy out there constructing an experimental cattle dip which would be much cheaper to build than the conventional plunge tank. More important still, this tank would also reduce by more than half the almost prohibitively high recurrent expenditure on the new insecticide, hexachlorethane, for the control of East Coast fever. Such was the need to economise on the cost of insecticides and other inputs which could otherwise easily exceed the market value of the local animals. The site for the trial was an extensive area of grassland to the south-east of the dense thorn bush which the groundnutters intended to clear but it was safe for the local cattle owners because of their grazing rights which were jealously guarded for them by the District Officer at Mpwapwa. It was ideal for the purpose because East Coast fever was endemic there and, as a result, a high proportion of the young stock succumbed to the disease during their first year of life. This accounted for the low stocking rate and the consequent abundance of grass throughout the whole year. It was also ideal for weekend breaks away from the relative confinement and proximity to work at Mpwapwa!

Beakbane had pitched his tent in the shade of a flat-topped Acacia tree on flat ground sloping gently down from the nearby hills. When we arrived on Friday afternoon a group of the local cattle owners were knocking off, having almost finished their task of bringing a supply of water to the site. This had been done over the previous few days by simply digging a narrow trench from the nearby hills along contours roughly marked out by Beakbane. They were a cheery lot, and while a tent was being erected for Jack and Kathleen, they chattered away enthusiastically about the prospects of having their own dip to protect their cattle from East Coast fever because, '*paka miaka mingi sana wanayama wingi wanakufa*' (for many years past many animals are dying). This was again typical of the cooperative relationship that existed between cattle-owning tribes and the Veterinary Department.

It was a self-catering outing and on the last night, even though Kathleen was a superb cook, I insisted on her taking it easy while I prepared the dinner. It turned out to be a gargantuan meal that finished up with plum pudding, of all things, topped off with sweetened condensed milk. Sated, we lay around the campfire until a late hour and eventually peeled off, one by one, to bed. Next morning we visited the Bains and on our return found everything packed away, so we were able to load up and get on our way. Up to that point, the switch-off had been one long laugh. Several miles along the road Ray, who was sitting in an armchair on the back of the lorry, banged on the top of the cab for me to stop. He looked ghastly but he thought that a little walk would help. Thereupon, he began to vomit and to our horror brought up what seemed to us to be a pint or two of blood and then fainted. He had been suffering from stomach trouble for some months past so we concluded that the haemorrhage was the result of a gastric ulcer. How I regretted my thoughtlessness in having served him with lamb chops, green peas and the Christmas pudding covered in sweetened condensed milk! We were all horrified, and there we were on a bumpy earth road some twenty-five miles away from Mpwapwa and the nearest clinic. Our first job was to fix up a camp bed with mattress and blankets on the back of the lorry. Somehow we managed to haul him on board. He was a little better by the time we got him into bed in his lonely bachelor's quarters with Dr Dikshit in attendance. Nothing much could be done for him at Mpwapwa, however, so he was sent on the hazardous journey by the next train to Dar es Salaam, 250 miles away. Fortunately, after a few weeks in hospital he was fit again and back to work.

Our relative isolation from medical facilities cut no ice with the older members of the department, such as CJ who even in the thirties had spent a good deal of his time on walking safaris in much more inaccessible parts of the country. In those circumstances the dread disease was blackwater fever, a frequently fatal complication of malaria in which the combined effect of the parasite and heavy doses of quinine caused a sudden disintegration of red blood corpuscles, thereby releasing haemoglobin into the blood stream from which it was excreted by the kidneys into the urine – hence the term blackwater. If this condition occurred while on safari, the only treatment, according to CJ, was for his companion or his boys to erect a tent over the patient because movement of any kind could be fatal. After that, the patient had to be given all the fluids he could take while a message was being sent to the nearest station where there were medical facilities, in the hope that the patient would not be dead before help arrived.

As I whiled away my time in Mpwapwa waiting for leave I was very undecided about whether or not I should make it my last tour. On the one hand, I was fascinated by Africa in general and Tanganyika in particular;

by the size of the country, the charm of its fascinating people, the multiplicity of problems waiting to be tackled, the sense that there was so much to be done and so few to do it, and the responsibilities that one was given. I knew I would miss it terribly. On the other hand, as each letter from home made me more and more conscious of the buzz going on in my parents' hospitable home, our wide circle of friends calling on my sister during her convalescence, preparations underway for the wedding, and friends of my brother and myself who had settled back in Dublin after the war very much in evidence. I seemed to be missing a lot and that brought back to me how disruptive life in the Colonial Service was for family, and here I was ready for married life. While vacillating I was determined that if I did come back it would be to the laboratory as a Veterinary Research Officer because laboratory based research was the career I wanted to embark on. If I came back to the laboratory as a Veterinary Officer I would be transferred to the field whenever the need arose. By then Bertie Lowe had retired and Willie Burns was Acting Director. I explained my decision to Willie and suggested that if I did come back as a Research Officer I should like my leave to be extended so that I could study for a Diploma in Bacteriology. Willie thought it was an excellent idea but left the final decision to the substantive Director, Neil Reid, who was at that point on his way back from home leave. Shortly thereafter, my leave papers came through and there was a wild rush to hand my house and some personal belongings to Beakbane, who had moved in with me, and put the rest in the Headquarters' stores pending the final outcome.

My marching orders were to get down to Dar in good time to board a plane on 25 June, the very day my sister was to be married in Dublin. By coincidence Neil Reid arrived back in Dar from leave while I was there. He was perfectly satisfied that I should come back to Mpwapwa as a Veterinary Research Officer and undertook to forward the recommendation to the Colonial Office without delay. He was much in favour of my taking further training but felt, however, that study leave should be deferred until the end of my next tour. This was good news and we both parted well satisfied.

I left Dar the following day on a brand new twenty-two-seater Vickers Viking, which in terms of size and luxury was state of the art for

1947. Despite that, the journey to England was to take three nights and four days compared with a flying time of eleven hours today. Most of the time we flew at ground speeds of about 175 mph and an altitude of 9,000 feet. None of the crew had been to Africa before, so they wanted to learn and see all they could. As a result a close, casual relationship developed between passengers and crew. For example, on the flight to Nairobi a herd of elephants was spotted, whereupon the pilot suddenly swooped down to what seemed to be a hundred feet or so above the herd which thundered ahead of us bringing up a cloud of dust as we flew past. Not having seen enough, the pilot did a U-turn and brought us back for another glimpse. It was probably the nearest that some of the passengers had been to an elephant outside a zoo. The first night was spent in the cool comfort of Nairobi.

Next morning we landed to refuel at Juba in the Sudan some forty miles north of the border with Uganda. It was a different Africa, very flat and oppressively hot. As we left the plane, a member of the crew explained that a minor fault had to be attended to in one of the engines and pointed us to a pleasant hotel nearby for a morning coffee. As the morning wore on we were regularly informed on progress until the Captain joined us and told us that the mechanic had dropped a spanner into the works. It would take time to retrieve it. He asked us to have a quick lunch so that we could leave as soon as possible, in any event not later than 2.30 p.m. because 'we cannot land at Khartoum after dark'. The time came and went and at 3 p.m., to our dismay, we were bundled into the plane which took off immediately. The sun was sinking depressingly low in the west as we approached a massive bank of black cloud to the north which was illuminated almost continuously by spectacular flashes of fork lightning. It was too high to fly over so it had to be circumnavigated and that took time while the light faded with the words 'one cannot land at Khartoum after dark' ringing in our ears. But the Captain proved himself wrong; he could and he did land shortly after dark! The Grand Hotel on the banks of the Nile was, of course, not air-conditioned in those days and the towel around the waist, which substituted for pyjamas, and the sheet on which I lay seemed to have been taken straight out of a hot oven. Our stop next morning for lunch and refuelling was at Wadi Halfa immediately south of the Egyptian border and nowadays on the shores of the man-made Aswan Dam. Apparently our cruising range was only about 700 miles. The next stop, merely for refuelling, was at El Adem, a small settlement near the coast a few miles from Tobruk. In that general area, as we flew at a few thousand feet above the desert, we could clearly see an extensive network of tracks in the sand, many of them sweeping in great circles, which presumably had been made by tanks and other vehicles during the desert battles. It was hard to believe that these marks had remained undisturbed by the wind for so long.

That night we were accommodated on the Island of Malta in shabby, abandoned army huts, overlooking the Naval Base, which by then were serving as a transit camp. It was the first indication we had of the limited progress that had been made during the past two years in the re-construction of Europe. While we were confined to the camp there was plenty of time to reflect on the bravery of the Maltese people and the British forces who had sustained the German blockade and the attendant air raids, thereby preserving the freedom of the George Cross Island for the Allies, right up to the invasion of Sicily in July 1942 and protecting it thereafter until the end of the war. My personal memories centred round two remarkable individuals both of whom, in common with many others, had been seriously touched before the war by the light-hearted charm and ready laugh of sister Anna. She was much loved but had remained fancy-free. The first of the two individuals was a handsome, persistent young Englishman living in Dublin who, almost unnoticed, spent progressively more time in our hospitable home than he did with Anna in the nearby tennis club. Having established cordial relations with the whole family, further progress would almost certainly have been made had the war not intervened. After the Battle of Britain he volunteered and joined the RAF and in due course was posted to the isolation of Malta. At some point during this period, the second individual, an intrepid Captain Pearson was keeping his eyes skinned for German bombers while ferrying high octane aero-fuel through the blockade to the RAF on Malta. Just before the outbreak of war he had been on leave in Dublin. He too had been captivated by my sister's charm and left with definite intentions but, with characteristic consideration for my sister, he allowed his intentions to remain undeclared until after the war. The final outcome was tinged with sadness. Our RAF friend survived throughout most of the siege but died of poliomyelitis shortly before the blockade was lifted - a tragic irony. The sea captain came out of the war unscathed and became my brother-in-law two days before my plane touched down on Malta!

On our last lap the following day we stopped at Marseilles and eventually landed at Blackbushe, a small airport in the south of England. As I drove up by coach to London on a sunny evening at the end of June, the greenness and the garden-like tidiness of the countryside contrasted vividly with the dry, unkempt, brown appearance of Tanganyika. I was also taken aback by the striking evidence that the war was over: carefree people, all in civvy clothes, enjoying a stroll in the gentle sunshine of the long summer evening, no cardboard boxes containing gas masks hanging from their shoulders; others out for a spin in pre-war cars, a few stuck at the roadside probably out of petrol. Later in the day, ensconced in my old favourite hotel, the Regent Palace off Piccadilly Circus, it dawned on me that the views through the windows were no longer obstructed by the criss-cross pattern of paper strips that were stuck on the panes during the war to prevent fragments of glass flying about in the event of a near-miss. The blackout curtains were also gone and Piccadilly Circus was ablaze with light. What a contrast it was after the blackout that I had left behind almost three years previously.

The euphoria that had been engendered by the sights and sounds of London persisted during the train journey to Holyhead and intensified on the passage across the Irish Sea when the Sugar Loaf mountain eventually appeared above the horizon. I had been primed for the excitement of meeting my family on the quayside at Dun Laoghaire by a friend's account of the rousing reception he had received from his family and friends when he arrived at Dun Laoghaire on his first leave. As the gap between the side of the Mail Boat and the pier narrowed gently, the passengers hanging over the rail on the upper deck peered down to the groups on the wharf, eager to identify their own friends. Suddenly an elderly lady and a gentleman, friends of my parents, began to wave enthusiastically at me, or so it seemed. I was deeply touched that they had taken so much trouble at that early hour to join the welcoming party. As I responded, I noticed that a young lady almost next to me began to wave equally enthusiastically - it was their daughter. I had not known until then that she was on board! What a fool I felt! Worse was to come when I discovered that there was not even a single member of my family on the pier. It was a sorry business edging past the happy groups that were embracing long-lost friends as I made my way to the boat train, which in those days waited on the pier. When the train eventually started, despite my disconsolate mood, I stood up and looked out the window to get a better view of a crowd standing at the level crossing a the entrance to the pier. For some reason they had not been allowed to pass the barrier. There to my delight was my brother waving like a windmill; on the spur of the moment, with no regard for the sensitivities of my fellow-passengers, I roared an earthy expletive used only by him and me to mark moments of intense astonishment. I had just time to see him dashing towards my father's elderly car which I had last seen up on blocks for the 'duration'. In what seemed no time we both arrived almost simultaneously at Westland Row Station. How incredibly short the journey seemed and how small everything else was after the wide expanses of Tanganyika. In no time we were home with my parents and some friends who had lingered on after the wedding. The subsequent meeting with my parents was just as moving though more restrained by the presence of wedding guests.

There was much to do and many old friends to see during the glorious summer of 1947 but by August it was time to think about the future. At end of the month I was offered an appointment as a Lecturer in Veterinary Parasitology at the Liverpool School of Tropical Medicine. Before accepting I obtained an interview with a personnel officer at the Colonial Office in London who, amongst other things, dealt with the recruitment and posting of veterinary staff. The interview got off to a bad start. He turned out to be a supercilious young gentleman and immediately took objection to my informing him that the Director of Veterinary Services had agreed that I should return from leave as a research officer. He explained that it was not his job to create vacancies for research officers for 'chappies' like me who were not prepared to rough it in bush like other young men. When I explained patiently that there had been vacancies for research officers and an education officer for several years at Mpwapwa, which the Colonial Office had been unable to fill, he condescendingly went though his card index cabinet. He suddenly exclaimed, 'By Jove, you are right laddie'. Unfortunately, he added that there would have to be interviews and 'all that sort of thing'. For me time had run out; I accepted the post at Liverpool and did not see Africa again for five years. Sadly, following the submission of my letter of resignation, it transpired that prior to my visit to London I had, in fact, been a Veterinary Research Officer for some weeks, my name having appeared as such in the Official Gazette. Bureaucracy was still alive and well at the Colonial Office!

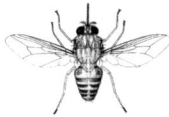

CHAPTER TWENTY-TWO

Africa Revisited

Life after Tanganyika. Return to Tanganyika thirty-one years later and the changes observed. Subsequently working over a period of 12 years until 1994 for the Irish Department of Foreign Affairs as Consultant for a livestock development project on the island of Pemba. Reflections on the early days of Independence and Nyerere's socialist policies. Later seeing the benefits of private enterprise.

After my brush with the personnel officer at the Colonial Office I suffered from homesickness for Africa during the next five years. I took up my appointment at Liverpool in September. My principal assignment was to lecture to the veterinary undergraduates of the University's Veterinary School which was located nearby but as I was deeply conscious of my own need for further training I looked forward to sitting at the feet of Professor R. M. Gordon who was a world authority on tropical parasitology. The Tropical School was a friendly place reflecting the warm, unaffected nature of Liverpudlians generally. However, life was still very austere in post-war England; consumer goods of all kinds were still in short supply and food rationing was as severe as ever. One of my lasting memories was of never having had quite enough food to stave off the cold damp of that Liverpool winter. How I longed for the warmth and the wide, open spaces of Tanganyika! Towards the end of the second term my health broke down and I was ordered prolonged sick leave which was readily granted but in the circumstances I felt obliged to relinquish my post.

After a prolonged convalescence I took up employment with the Irish Department of Agriculture. I was specifically recruited to develop programmes for the control of parasitic diseases of farm animals as part of a scheme funded by the Marshall Plan for European Recovery. My first assignment was to travel extensively for six months in the USA studying recent developments in veterinary parasitology at laboratories of the Federal Department of Agriculture and in several universities. On my return to Ireland my report was accepted but I was retained at Headquarters for an interminable time waiting for laboratory facilities which by 1952 had not been provided.

In 1952, after almost two incredibly frustrating years, two developments occurred which changed the whole course of my life. The first began with the receipt of a letter from my old friend Jack Wilde. He was on leave of absence in England in the process of being transferred from Mpwapwa to take up an appointment as Director of Veterinary Laboratory Services for the Federal Government of Nigeria at Vom on the Bauchi Plateau, some 500 miles north of Lagos. Having satisfied myself that there was still no assurance that I would be provided with the necessary laboratory facilities in Ireland within the foreseeable future, I jumped at the opportunities actually waiting for me in Nigeria. By May 1952 my resignation had been accepted by the Irish Department of Agriculture and my appointment had been confirmed by the Colonial Office in London.

Almost immediately, while I was doing my last job for the Department of Agriculture at the Royal Dublin Society's Spring Show at Ballsbridge, I met and fell in love with Joyce Wright, a stunning little redhead several years younger than me who I soon learnt faced all the little problems in life with her ready smile followed by practical action. During the rest of that month the courtship was almost continuous because Joyce was to sail from Cobh early in June for three months in America and I was already booked to sail from Liverpool to Lagos in July. Shortly before her departure I was greatly encouraged when she casually invited me, as we happened to pass the Abbey Theatre, to accompany her inside to meet her father, Dossie Wright, who I subsequently learnt had been a member of the Abbey since the early days of Yeats and Lady Gregory. At the end of a rather brief conversation with him I was further encouraged by the seemingly knowing smile he bestowed on both of us as we withdrew. After that it seemed the most natural thing for me to drive Joyce to Cobh to see her safely on board the Mauretania. It was a touching farewell that immediately initiated a regular correspondence that increased in frequency and warmth during the following eighteen months.

Vom turned out to be another veterinary enclave, considerably larger than Mpwapwa. In addition to the extensive laboratories of the Federal Veterinary Department it also housed laboratories of the West African Institute for Trypanosomiasis. Situated on the Bauchi Plateau, some 5,000 feet above sea level, the climate was pleasantly cool for most of the year. The expatriate staff of the two institutions and their partners, excluding children, generally numbered about fifty. Consequently the social and physical infrastructure was much more suitable for the family life of Europeans than that of Mpwapwa only five years previously, so I had no hesitation in increasing the frequency of letter writing to Joyce. Better still, the accelerated rate was reciprocated in Dublin. The work was also immensely satisfying. During my first tour of eighteen months I travelled extensively throughout Nigeria organising surveys to determine the parasitic diseases of major economic importance in cattle, sheep and goats in representative ecological areas. From this programme a research programme emerged which required the services of a greatly increased staff. Fortunately the necessary funding was provided to the extent that by 1956 it became necessary to develop an Animal Production Division with a staff of six scientific officers, two farm managers and supporting technicians. The Division concerned itself mainly with diseases of impaired productivity, animal husbandry, breeding and genetics.

By the end of my first tour I was more than satisfied that Vom was an excellent place for married life. As far as I was concerned it would not be for want of asking if I were to return from leave as a bachelor. This resolve became progressively stronger during the fourteen days' voyage from Lagos to Liverpool. Within two weeks of my arriving home we were engaged and were subsequently married in Dublin almost exactly two years after our meeting at the Spring Show. Joyce settled into Vom comfortably and to my great pleasure greatly enjoyed accompanying me in the early years to the remote parts of Nigeria to which my work took me.

After Independence, which was granted in 1960, several expatriate members of my own staff decided to leave because there was no longer promotion prospects for non-Nigerians. In 1961 I followed suit in order to take up a position as the Statutory Lecturer of Parasitology, University College Dublin (UCD), at the Veterinary College at Ballsbridge. The

previous year a bizarre change in the arrangements for veterinary education in Ireland had been put in place by the Government which
involved establishing two autonomous veterinary schools in the premises
of the Veterinary College of Ireland, one belonging to Trinity College
Dublin (TCD) and the other to University College Dublin. (For further
reading see Donnelly, W.T.C. and Monaghan, M.L. (2001).) Six years
later I was appointed to the Chair of Clinical Veterinary Sciences in TCD
and subsequently became Director and then Dean of the Faculty. My
administrative duties left me with little time for extra-curricular activities
though I did manage to visit Nigeria on three successive occasions as
external examiner for the University of Nigeria.

In 1977 the veterinary schools of TCD and UCD were amalgamat-
ed within UCD. As a result I became Professor and Head of its new
Department of Veterinary Parasitology. With more time at my disposal I
returned regularly to Africa for brief assignments in the Sudan, Uganda,
Tanzania and Zambia. Following several visits to Zambia I was invited by
the Irish Department of Foreign Affairs to serve as Inaugural Dean of a
new School of Veterinary Medicine in the University of Zambia at
Lusaka which was about to be built by the Japanese International
Cooperation Agency (JICA) at a cost of 23 million US dollars. Though
my post there, and those of some other colleagues, was funded by the
Irish Government, I was also required to serve as the Advisor to JICA's
Veterinary Education Project in setting up the academic structures and
courses in the new school. I arrived in Lusaka just before the first class was
admitted to the first year of veterinary studies which was conducted in
rather unsatisfactory accommodation in the School of Mines. At that
point the academic staff consisted of only three veterinary lecturers
supported by an excellent laboratory technician from Bristol. I was immediately thrown into the task of trying to recruit academics, including short
term visiting lecturers, and technicians from all over the world, including
Africa, Japan, Ireland, Great Britain and from European countries on both
sides of the Iron Curtain. It was hoped that I would have completed the
recruiting process in time for the commencement of the courses of the
first and subsequent veterinary years. It was a nerve-racking business that
continued unabated for the remainder of my term of office. However,
our stay in Zambia was a wonderful experience for both me and my wife,

due largely to the competence, charm and warmth of the Japanese personnel.

When I arrived only the foundations of the elegant buildings had been laid but even then several large containers were in place on the periphery of the extensive site. These had been brought by sea from Japan to Dar es Salaam and thence by rail through Tanzania and Zambia to Lusaka. They contained materials and equipment unobtainable in Zambia which were required during the first phase of the building operations. More containers continued to arrive until there was a veritable circular stockade of numbered containers encircling the whole site. As successive containers were opened they were unfailingly found to contain the material required for the next phase. By the time the building operations had been completed the remaining containers were opened to reveal all manner of laboratory equipment such as microscopes, centrifuges, incubators and autoclaves. By the time the building operations had been completed the remaining containers were opened to reveal all manner of laboratory and hospital equipment such as microscopes, centrifuges, incubators, autoclaves, operating tables, surgical instruments and anaesthetic equipment. Teaching aids such as cameras, projectors, photocopiers, and a full range of office equipment were also included. The most impressive feature of the whole operation was the fact that the fully equipped complex was officially handed over to the University on the precise date promised in March 1986, only two years after the first foundations were laid. The adherence to the promised date was almost certainly a record for any development project undertaken by any aid agency in Zambia.

The warm relations that I enjoyed with my Japanese colleagues, and indeed with other colleagues of many different nationalities, and which Joyce enjoyed with their wives, more than compensated for the inevitable frustrations that occurred constantly at work and at home. We were able to share some of this truly wonderful experience with our family, who were by then grown up. Andrew and his wife Joyce, and our daughters Anna and Juliet managed to visit us in Lusaka on holiday

However, believing as I did in the virtues of low-tech aid projects, I could not avoid worrying from time to time about the possibility that the sophisticated facilities, which so many donors had helped to provide, might prove unsustainable in the long term. I was particularly conscious of the problems of sustainability because during my time at Lusaka I was also engaged as Technical Consultant to a highly practical Irish project involved in livestock improvement on the island of Pemba in Tanzania. The project aimed to improve the welfare of smallholders by the application of relatively simple technology in the fields of veterinary medicine and animal husbandry accompanied by word of mouth instruction. In comparison it seemed a safer, more sustainable approach in the economic circumstances of the time. To explain this more fully it is necessary to take the reader back to my first visit to the new country of Tanzania in 1978 (almost thirty-one years after my leisurely flight home from Tanganyika) when I was a member of a delegation funded by the Irish Department of Foreign Affairs. The purpose of the visit was to ascertain how resources available to Higher Education in Ireland might assist the development of universities and technical colleges in Tanzania and Zambia.

Not only was the country different in name to the one I had left, it was now an independent nation under the socialist government of President Nyerere. When Independence came in 1961 Julius Nyerere, Chairman of the Tanganyika African National Union (TANU), became President. He was a highly intelligent idealist who had worked for the previous fifteen years to win the freedom of his native land by constitutional means. By the time independence arrived he had gained the support and the blessing of the European settlers as well as the moral and financial support of the western world. Unfortunately, his misguided idealism led him to pursue a mixture of the socialism of China and that of the Soviet Union. It did not take long for me to perceive the extent to which socialism had taken hold and impoverished the country during seventeen years of self-government.

We arrived at Dar es Salaam's impressive international airport, which had probably been built by some of the overseas aid that had been pouring into the country since Independence. As soon as we reclaimed our luggage, we were surrounded by a surplus of poorly clad porters all clamouring to carry our bags. At various checkpoints we were addressed by dispirited officials as *Ndugu*, meaning brother or comrade. We were then waved away to fill up multiple copies of voluminous forms relating to customs, emigration, currency and health. One got the impression that a variety of consultants from an overseas aid agency had set up systems everywhere for the compilation of statistics that would fill offices and would seldom, if ever, be used again. The experience at the airport was the first indication to the visitor that bureaucracy had become a way of life for many and was in the process of strangling the country.

Nevertheless, the currency forms at the airport had to be taken seriously because all those arriving from overseas were required to declare the foreign currency in their possession and to obtain receipts for all sums converted into local currency while in the country. All such receipts had to be retained for inspection before departure to show that no illegal transactions had taken place. The official exchange rate of Tanzanian Shilling for hard currencies was so low compared with the black market rates that extreme measures had to be taken to protect the official, unrealistic rate. Even the identification numbers on saleable articles such as cameras had to be entered on an appropriate form to satisfy customs officials that departing visitors had not traded them for bundles of Tanzanian Shillings.

Dar es Salaam itself had a run-down appearance compared to what I had known. The once sparklingly white two-story buildings on Acacia Avenue looked crumbly and in dire need of paint. There was no sign of the much-loved New Africa Hotel with its red tiled roof and mosquito-netted beds on the open verandas. Only the name, not the character, had been preserved in a new, rectangular office-block-like structure. The trim lawns of the bungalows on the way to Oyster Bay, which had formerly been occupied by European officials, were now overgrown and the ayahs in their spotlessly white overalls pushing the prams were nowhere to be seen. Fortunately, we did not have to stay in the hot, lifeless atmosphere of a hotel bedroom in the centre of Dar. Our Embassy had booked us into a beach holiday motel some ten miles to the north at the end of an incredibly bumpy road. It was hard to know whether the heavily pot-holed tarmac stretches along which the Embassy Land Rover juddered were any better than the equally bumpy but less juddery, old-fashioned earth roads.

The journey proved to be well worth the discomfort. The hotel, which had been built by an Israeli company, was situated on its own delightful beach overlooking the Indian Ocean with individual chalets located in the much needed shade of a mature coconut plantation adjacent to the central facilities; namely offices, bar, restaurant and swimming pool. It had been built as a holiday resort for the express purpose of attracting tourists and their precious hard currency from overseas. The only ingredient missing was tourists who presumably had found the services and the cost of the Mombasa beaches better value and perhaps less hazardous than the risk of falling coconuts referred to on warning notices along the pathways. Consequently, our beach resort was occupied largely by aid workers like ourselves whose philanthropy was rewarded by superb lobster thermador and other delicacies at the expense of their own taxpayers. Here again, and throughout the whole of Tanzania, the scarcity of hard currency was the name of the game; all accounts of non-residents had to be paid in hard currency, at five-star rates, and any change due was given in Tanzanian Shillings. Such transactions, here and elsewhere in Africa, were attended by resounding bangs of the ubiquitous rubber stamps. It was such a liberating sound when transacting business in government departments, banks and especially in the departures hall at the airport as one sweated in the struggle at currency desks, health checks, customs and, above all, emigration before boarding the plane.

During our visit such matters were fascinating for my four companions on their first visit to Tanzania. But for me it was bliss to discover that I could still speak Kiswahili after a fashion and, in doing so, I found that the charm and the inimitable sense of humour of most of those with whom I came in contact at the hotel, and elsewhere in Tanganyika, was still intact after so many years of deprivation.

On our way into Dar es Salaam early one morning we found that soldiers and, to a lesser extent, the police did not fit into the above generalisation. We had a mid-morning appointment with the Minister for Education but the leader of our delegation had not adapted himself to the lack of urgency that attended the execution of almost any task. He certainly had not heard the Swahili proverb 'haraka, haraka, haina baraka' (hurry, hurry, has no blessing) or for that matter 'poli, poli, kamata mtumbili' (slowly, slowly, catch the monkey). Consequently, he became progressively more agitated when the Embassy Land Rover failed to arrive. Eventually, we managed to hire a ramshackle taxi, devoid of shock absorbers, which sank lower and lower onto its springs as each of us, bent double, squeezed in. A few miles down the road, as we passed an army encampment, a loud bang rang out in our immediate vicinity which, to our relief, turned out to be no more deadly than a puncture. To the consternation of us all, the driver with a '*tabu sana*' (big trouble) sheepishly informed us that he had no spare wheel. The leader of our group, distraught at the prospect of being late for the Minister, announced that he was going to make a phone call from the army camp. I pointed out that a large notice, roughly translated, read ENTRY STRICTLY PROHIBITED. With my experience of other African countries, I pleaded with him not to go in, but to no avail. As soon as he went in he was arrested and marched away at gunpoint. My companions were disappointed when I refused to follow him; instead I negotiated across the fence with those remaining in the guard room, dropping the words 'Irish Embassy' at every possible opportunity. Eventually word was taken back to wherever our colleague was being held and, in due course, he reappeared, still at gunpoint, and rather miffed that those who had accused him of spying were not impressed that we were merely trying to assist their University.

Our time in Dar es Salaam was taken up with visits to the relevant Government Departments and, of course, with senior officials at the University of Dar es Salaam, at that time, the only university in the country. The latter was located on a delightful, well cared for site on relatively high ground looking across a flat coastal plain to Dar es Salaam in the distance with glimpses of the Indian Ocean beyond. The elegant Campus (see illust.), which had been built by generous overseas aid, was indeed a thing of beauty but not an unqualified joy for ever, the main problem once again being lack of hard currency for recurrent expenditure. This problem was brought home vividly to the members of the delegation during our onward journey to the University's Agricultural and Veterinary Campus which was situated at Morogoro, a hundred miles inland from Dar es Salaam. We were provided with a Land Rover and a driver by the University for the journey and when we called at the transport yard for fuel we learnt that most of the other vehicles parked there were grounded for lack of spare parts. We made good speed along an excellent tarmac road en route to Morogoro until we had yet another blow-out. This time we had a fine spare wheel but no jack! Even though two members of our team were distinguished engineers there was no need for high technology. All the driver needed of the engineers was muscle with which to lift the vehicle onto precariously-balanced rocks; then the academics stood and watched. (See illust.) This could have been a lesson for many of aid agencies at the beginning; start off with low technology and work up.

The fundamental problem at the Veterinary School at Morogoro was the same, namely reasonably good physical facilities but an acute shortage of funds for recurrent expenditure. The campus was located on the lower slopes of the majestic Uluguru Mountains surrounded by its own lush farmland. As one passed through the front gates and continued along the gentle incline to the main buildings, the sight of a large herd of pedigree Jersey cows grazing contentedly in the cool of the evening was delightful to behold. The herd had been donated by the New Zealand Government and transported some 8,000 miles across the Southern and Indian Oceans. This was a real agricultural campus complete with proper farm buildings, including a veterinary clinic staffed by a competent African Veterinary Assistant trained by the former regime, a fine cattle dip, the exotic Jersey cows, plenty of the local Zebu cattle, lots of goats and some sheep. The buildings for the School of Agriculture were already in place as were the assembly hall, student accommodation, attractive staff houses and a guesthouse complete with bar which doubled as a staff common room and overnight accommodation for visitors. The building of the Veterinary School, which was part of a Danish aid project, was nearing completion and bright, well-motivated students were already receiving instruction from well-qualified Tanzanian academics who would be supported, in due course, by visiting professors, lecturers and technicians from Denmark, Ireland and elsewhere. In general, the prospects were good that the School would be capable of producing competent veterinary graduates. The tragedy was that the country was broke to such an extent that devaluation of the Tanzanian Shilling had fallen so low that competent university lecturers, with hard-earned higher degrees in their specialised fields, were reduced to running little businesses, such as poultry farming in their own compounds, to supplement their almost meaningless salaries.

As I saw more and more of the country in the succeeding years it was depressing to encounter the frustration that bright young graduates experienced in trying to practise their profession in the failed socialist society. As private enterprise had been abolished there was no possibility of engaging in private practice. Moreover, Nyerere's ujamaa scheme, an extreme form of agrarian socialism that had involved moving smallholders into larger settlements in order to engage in collective farming, had failed. Before this scheme, the established way of life outside the relatively few townships was subsistence farming which verged on private ownership supplemented by voluntary sharing. Within this system each family built its own house, usually with the assistance of neighbours, and was allocated a patch of land or *shamba* nearby. The cultivation, weeding and harvesting of the *shamba* was conducted by the household, generally assisted by members of the extended family, with the men taking the lesser share of the work. Water was fetched by the women, often from considerable distances, and any surplus produce was carried, again by the women, to the nearest market where the proceeds were used to purchase simple commodities such as salt, soap, *kitambas* and other clothing. Such expeditions were part of the social life. Ujamaa aimed to bring families in from their scattered villages and smallholdings to larger settlements provided with clinics, schools, piped water and communal land. Life there was to be coordinated by a member or members of the revolutionary party, Chama cha Mapinduzi (CCM) which was by then not just the ruling political party but the Government itself. In due course, these designated local members became the eyes and ears of the party, not merely co-ordinators. As time went on private enterprise was abolished, banks and insurance companies were nationalised, ownership of property and renting of houses was discouraged and a variety of semi-state bodies were set up for a whole range of activities such as distribution of agricultural inputs, purchasing and marketing of agricultural products, management of dairy farms and ranches and such manufacturing as had been done previously by private companies.

Ujamaa failed to achieve its goals of collective farming. Many smallholders resisted being uprooted from their established way of life and those who were persuaded to move, or forced to do so by the local CCM officials of the ruling party, did not take kindly to collectivisation. For example, in the absence of transport they had to endure the hardship of having to walk miles to the outlying fields. This was particularly resented by the men who traditionally expected their wives to do more than their fair share of the cultivation. Instead of earning cash for the sale of their produce, with which the smallholders had previously purchased the necessities of life, including simple agricultural inputs, they were rewarded instead with coupons to exchange at their so-called co-operatives. The latter, like their counterparts that had replaced private enterprise in other fields, were crippled by bureaucracy and had little, if any, cash for the purchase of commodities required by the collective farmers.

Had the ujamaa resettlements been economically successful they would, no doubt, have provided an outlet for the employment of veterinary graduates in clinical practice. But they were not and consequently, most of the veterinary graduates were destined to end up as veterinary officers in central government where they were confined for most of the time to their offices through lack of transport and other basic facilities.

★

I revisited Mpwpawa several years later. By then the headquarters and the laboratories of the Veterinary Department had been transferred to Dar es Salaam and all that remained of the veterinary presence was a diagnostic laboratory cum clinic located in the erstwhile bustling headquarters building. On that occasion the staff were practically idle and frustrated beyond measure because of the shortage of equipment, laboratory reagents and drugs. Only the monkeys had been unaffected by the changes that had taken place since my departure in 1947; there they were, a later generation rampaging across the tin roof of the building just as their forebears had been doing so many years previously.

Across the river, on the way up to the laboratories it was depressing to see that the once trim golf course had been built over by a sprawl of uninspiring, single-storey classrooms and dormitories of a training school. It was, however, a comfort to find that the actual buildings of the laboratories, which had been used for veterinary research and vaccine production, first by the Germans and then by the British, from 1905 onwards, were still intact and easily identified. At the time of my visit the buildings housed a Livestock Production Research Institute which conducted, as best it could with the meagre funds available, research and extension work into

Ugogo involving livestock breeding, nutrition, husbandry and pasture improvement. I was received with great courtesy by the enthusiastic Director, Dr Daz. He had faithfully recorded the names of most of the Directors and Chief Veterinary Research Officers for the period 1922 to 1961 and was hungry for biographical information relating to them. During a conducted tour of the premises he was delighted to assist me in identifying the various buildings and to learn about the uses to which they had been put. Sadly, the life that I had known and enjoyed so much in the forties was gone for ever and as I recognised the houses of my old friends it was sad to accept that not even their ghosts, far less any of their offspring, had remained. They had long since taken themselves and their genes to cooler climes. This sense of loss eased a little when Dr Daz proudly showed me a herd of 140 dairy cows that he referred to as members of the Mpwapwa breed. He assured me that some of them had the same genes as those that CJ had selected and nurtured with equal pride almost forty years previously.

It became noticeable to me that Tanzania began to change for the better in 1986 by which time many of Mr Nyerere's followers were openly disillusioned by his form of socialism. At that point he handed over the presidency to Mr Mwinyi, though he retained considerable power by remaining Chairman of the revolutionary party. With the assistance of loans from the International Monetary Fund, the new president began to restore private enterprise by bringing the official rate for the Tanzanian Shilling progressively nearer the more realistic rate at which it changed hands on the black market. This freed up the market. As a result traders and other entrepreneurs, instead of the incompetent State corporations which by then were being disbanded, gained access to foreign currency for the importation of capital equipment and consumer goods. The appearance of consumer goods in the shops boosted the morale of the general population and gave them the incentive to work for more, an incentive that they had never had till then.

★

I had the opportunity during regular visits to the island of Pemba during the period 1982 to 1994 to see the changes that unfolded there during the transition from state-control to private enterprise. The island, which is 67 km long by 22 km at the widest point on the much-indented coastline, lies 40 km north of Zanzibar and some 65 km east of Tanga on the mainland. In 1982, with a rapidly rising human population it was already the most densely populated rural area of Tanzania and despite the fact that many of its smallholder farmers between them owned some 65,000 head of cattle these animals contributed little produce for human consumption. The pressure of the growing human population on the available arable land was increasing progressively so there was clearly a need for the introduction of more efficient, intensive methods of livestock production. Consequently, in 1982, the Irish Department of Foreign Affairs undertook to assist the Government of Zanzibar (which was responsible for the administration of Pemba within the Union) in its endeavours.

There was already a herd of Jersey cows on a government dairy farm which were dipped every week. Dipping significantly reduced deaths from East Coast fever but the management of the farm was strangled by bureaucracy with the result that milk yields were disappointingly low for such a breed and the morbidity and mortality rates of calves and other young stock were high. There was obviously no point in wasting precious hard currency in trying to support this type of enterprise so at an early stage it was decided to concentrate on smallholders who in the tradition of the island virtually owned or had rights to patches of land amounting in most cases to about two acres. Most of the smallholders kept two to four head of cattle which were grazed on fallow land and tethered to protect the adjoining crops of maize, sweet potatoes, yams, and bananas.

Between 1982 and 1986 the project got underway with the collection of information from surveys with which to devise possible means of improving the traditional farming system. Because of the scarcity of foreign currency life was difficult on the island. There was practically nothing, other than local produce, to be purchased on Pemba. Even soap made from the oil of the coconut palms, which were everywhere to be seen, was almost unobtainable. There was a modern hospital in Wete but most of the time it was short of quite basic medicines and other materials. The school children at the Fidel Castro School often had no writing paper or even chalk for their slates. Consequently, practically all the material required for the project, such as laboratory equipment, veterinary medicines, instruments, motor cycles and bicycles had to be acquired by the slow process of importing them from Ireland. The few materials that were manufactured on the mainland, such as cement and fencing wire, had to be paid for in hard currency.

Two hotels had been built on the island, one in Chake Chake and the other in Wete, the two small towns on the island. They had been built in anticipation of attracting tourists but both were almost invariably empty. The bedrooms on the first floor of the hotel at Chake Chake, where the first Project Leader, John Griffin, and I stayed on a preliminary visit in 1982, had wash-hand basins but piped water only reached the hotel intermittently because of the shortage of diesel for the pump at the town's reservoir. The resourceful hotel manager had tried to minimise the inconvenience by resorting to low technology. This consisted of installing a galvanised water tank halfway up the stairs. A garden hose, just long enough to reach the tank, was fed through the dining room from an out-door tap. In order to give the water the necessary lift from the dining room to the stairs it was threaded over a dining room chair standing on one of the many redundant tables. To bridge the gap between the tank and the guest's wash-hand basin, the water was carried onwards in buckets one of which was provided for each guest. A weakness here was that the plugs for the spanking white basins were missing so one had to use a mug for shaving, then stuff a handkerchief into the plug hole and wash as quickly as possible before the water drained away. Another fault in the system was that the pumps at the reservoir came on at unpredictable times, generally while all of the staff were out, which was most of the time. On returning to the hotel one was liable to find the tank overflowing with a cascade of water tumbling down the stairs, across the foyer and out through the front door which was always open. On the first few occasions when this happened, John and I tended to panic but nobody else seemed to share our concern. Subsequently, we too became so accustomed to the arrangement that on those occasions when we returned to the hotel, hot and sticky after a day's work, and found a waterfall in full spate our immediate reaction was to acknowledge the refreshing cascade with the comment 'Oh good, the water's on again!'

This then was the state of the infrastructure between 1982 and 1986 while the project was feeling its way by trial and error to introduce improvements. One of the worries during this period was whether a sufficient number of smallholders would be prepared to make the necessary effort to cooperate. I also had grave doubts as to whether the fundamental concept of the project was flawed and was also concerned that our expectations were perhaps unrealistic. Were we just throwing Irish taxpayers' money away? Therefore, it was comforting on one of my visits to see how well one of the experimental units which had been provided with a pure-bred Jersey cow was being managed and to contemplate the potential benefits it could have for the social life of the villages. At the end of a day's work I set off for a quiet stroll to one of the experimental units and, as invariably happens on such occasions, I was followed by a group of lively youngsters whose numbers kept increasing as we progressed. On arrival at our destination we found the owner's ten-year-old son solemnly preparing for the evening milking of the solitary cow. He had already washed and scrubbed the concrete floor and had filled the manger where the cow was chewing contentedly. There was no communication between him and the rest of us as he expertly tied the cow's tail to one of her legs. He then carefully measured the required quantity of disinfectant, poured it into a gourd and set to washing the cow's udder. As the milk began to flow in a steady stream raising a froth in the bucket it was reassuring to see something being created from virtually nothing, not only for this boy's family but also for their customers. In contrast, my admittedly happy band of followers had nothing to do but mess around until the following morning when they set off on their long walk to the Fidel Castro School which had its own problems to cope with.

Despite my initial worries, the behaviour of the efficient little boy that I had encountered at the experimental unit proved to be unexceptional. As it transpired, the entrepreneurship and enthusiasm of the smallholders and counterpart officials proved to be quite remarkable, particularly after 1986 when private enterprise began to replace socialism as the official policy.

One of the overriding problems limiting milk production was East Coast fever which was endemic and widespread throughout the island. The disease was one hundred per cent fatal to exotic stock unless they were confined to a hopefully tick-free enclosure and sprayed once or twice a week with prohibitively expensive insecticides. In contrast the indigenous dwarf Zebu cattle possessed a highly effective innate resistance to the disease, having been exposed over untold generations to infected ticks. Unfortunately, the productivity of these small cows was so low that they were kept mainly for prestige or for slaughter on festive occasions such as weddings and funerals.

Eventually, after much trial and error, the project adopted an approach that became known as the Improved Traditional Livestock Management System (ITLM System). The first problem to be overcome was the low productivity of the indigenous dwarf Zebu cattle. These small cows were slow to mature and when they eventually reached breeding age they calved only every second year and seldom produced more than a litre of milk per day. Consequently, it was decided to inseminate the cows of the cooperating smallholders with Jersey semen. Frozen semen was brought from as far afield as New Zealand and Ireland to Pemba where it was stored in liquid nitrogen. Local young men were trained in the technique of artificial insemination and when called they carried the semen to the smallholdings in thermos flasks either by bicycle or motor bike, depending on the distance. Concurrently, extension officers were being trained in the basics of veterinary medicine, animal husbandry and nutrition in preparation for the care of the more highly productive half-bred calves.

The next problem that had to be faced, one on which the success of the whole undertaking depended, was the susceptibility of half-bred Jerseys to East Coast fever. The imperfect techniques available at the time (and to this day) for artificial immunisation were tried and proved impracticable for use on Pemba, so a 'natural' method of immunising the half-breds was devised which, thanks to the diligence and competence of the smallholders and the extension officers, proved effective. The procedure involved tethering the half-bred calves, from birth onwards, with their dams on natural grazing. The rainfall pattern on Pemba ensured that ticks were active throughout the year. As a result, practically all of the calves thus exposed became infected during the first few weeks or months of life. During this period they were kept under scrutiny by the owners, all of whom were well able to recognise the first symptoms of ECF. At the first sign, they notified their extension officer who came immediately by bicycle and treated the infected calf with a new drug which, fortuitously, had just come on the market. Those that survived the first infection (some eighty to ninety per cent) developed an immunity that was subsequently boosted and maintained throughout the rest of their lives by continued exposure to infection.

The half-bred calves and cows required, at least, twice as much nutrition as the local Zebus to enable them to express their full production potential. This was provided by supplementing the limited grazing with a wide variety of crop residues such as the leaves of sweet potatoes, cassava, cow peas, groundnuts, pawpaws and banana palms. Kitchen waste including banana, mango, pawpaw, and lemon skins and the fleshy pith of jack-fruit and bread-fruit (given by neighbours in expectation of a little milk when a child was ill) was also used. The supplementary protein required by high yielding cows was provided by feeding the leaves of nitrogen-rich leguminous shrubs, some of which were grown as hedges. Another nitrogen-rich supplement was the residue of coconuts after extraction of the oil by the housewife for cooking. Here it may be of interest to note that the design of the project was based largely on the simple fact that ruminants, in contrast to humans, are capable of digesting cellulose thereby converting some of the released energy into milk and meat. Consequently, there was little competition between the ruminants and the rapidly rising human population of the island. Needless to say, cooperating smallholders required considerable instruction in the husbandry and feeding of their half-bred stock right through from calving to milk production. Initially this was done on a one-to-one basis until a number of units had been established. Thereafter, groups were taken to the best of the established units where instruction was given by the Extension Officers by word of mouth. The instruction was of a highly practical nature. In this context, each Extension Officer was encouraged to set up and manage his own unit so that his considerable theoretical knowledge was augmented by practical experience.

The growth rate of the half-bred calves proved to be very satis-factory. They came into heat much sooner than their Zebu dams and con-sequently began their first lactation proportionately earlier. In preparation for the latter each smallholder built a simple open-sided shelter with thatched roof and a concrete floor. The framework was made from locally grown bush poles so there was little need for hard currency. The purpose of the shelter was to provide comfort during the rains and also to enable the cow to be tied up during milking while contentedly chewing her supplementary rations. Where possible, everything was low technology. For example, daily milk yields were measured and recorded on a pad that was simply stuffed into the thatch until collected by the extension officer. Likewise, a small supplement of calcium diphosphate for every litre of milk produced had to be sprinkled on the feed. This was dispensed not in grams but in so many matchbox fills.

When a sufficient number of cows had completed their first lactations, milk yields proved to be very satisfactory - in most cases considerably more than six litres per cow per day, the latter being approximately six times that of the local Zebu cows. But the most satisfactory feature of the project was the enthusiasm, the initiative, and the entrepreneurship of the majority of the smallholders when they were empowered to make their own decisions and manage their own affairs, entirely free from the constraints of state control. The resourcefulness of one landless young man who wished to set up his own unit is illustrated in Plate X. He managed to acquire a half-bred heifer which he grazed on a vacant, grassy patch of land attached to a Government office. He was not allowed to erect the recommended thatched shelter on Government property so he improvised by erecting a temporary structure, complete with cantilevered roof, made from concrete blocks and corrugated iron sheets that were lying around.

Another enterprising, landless gentleman kept a half-bred cow in the middle of Chake Chake beside the vegetable market. (See illust.) She had access to limited grazing but her main fodder consisted of discarded vegetables of which there was an abundant supply next door. With the help of a little concentrate meal, containing protein-rich coconut cake imported from the mainland, she managed to produce nineteen litres a day at the height of her second lactation. As her first bull calf was a three-quarter-bred Jersey he was retained by the project for use as a stud bull. Having been successfully treated early in calfhood for naturally acquired ECF while still sucking his dam and subsequently exposed continuously to infected ticks he remained solidly immune to the disease for life. Consequently, he was able to wander around the villages with impunity whereas animals confined to concrete-floored pens under zero grazing systems remain susceptible for the rest of their lives. In the event of their being infected in adult life, for example, by ticks brought in on cut grass they would almost certainly die because the cost of medication for animals other than calves was prohibitive.

A disadvantage of being completely dependant on artificial insemination was the unreliability in the supply of liquid nitrogen that was imported from Zanzibar for the storage and transport of semen. Therefore, in the interest of sustainability, cooperating smallholders in localities where there were a number of units within walking distance of each other were encouraged to provide themselves with the services of a communal bull. (See illust.)

The social relationships between expatriate aid workers and Africans had changed completely since I had worked so many years previously as a Colonial Officer in Tanganyika. House servants and the locals generally were no longer 'boys', to be addressed by first name. Instead, they were afforded the title 'Mr'. During my second visit to Pemba I was struck by the warm relationship that had developed between the Project Leader and the first smallholder, Mr Ali Abdullah, who had been provided with a pure bred Jersey cow from the Government Dairy Farm to set up an experimental smallholding. The unit was close to the rather decrepit house in which the John and his intrepid young wife and their baby lived. In the cool of my first evening the smallholder appeared at the door and announced his presence with the conventional '*Hodi* Mr John?' ('May I come in Mr John?') This was followed by John's reply from behind the tattered mosquito gauze, '*Jambo* Mr Ali, *karibu*', ('Hello Mr Ali, do come in'). It was the first time I had heard Swahili spoken with a Cork accent and, as the days passed by, pleasantly punctuated by Mr Ali's evening visits accompanied by cups of tea, I began to think that I could just detect a slight Cork accent in Mr Ali's Swahili!

Livestock projects of this kind are slow to develop because of the time it takes for each new farmer to become established within the scheme. For example, by the time a new entrant's Zebu cow is inseminated almost four years elapses before her half-bred heifer is inseminated and subsequently comes into her first lactation. The cycle takes longer if the first calf turns out to be a male. Nevertheless, the Irish Department of Foreign Affairs stood by the project and continued to provide expatriate staff until 1995 when the management was handed over to a Pemban. There was every likelihood that the project would become sustainable but, even at worst, the welfare of the cooperating smallholders had been greatly improved and the knowledge and experience they had gained was being passed on to their children and would probably go, through them, to the next generation. Two years later, the number of cooperating smallholders had risen to 883; the smallholders were selling their surplus milk at a handsome profit at centres in Chake Chake and Wete. Private entrepreneurs were also making a little on the side by distributing milk by bicycle. Even ice cream was available from time to time in Wete!

The economic benefits and improvement in the lives of the ordinary people resulting from the introduction of private enterprise, following twenty-five years of socialism, became more and more evident on Pemba, Zanzibar and the mainland with the passage of each year. For example, the journey from Dar es Salaam to Zanzibar which had previously involved an infrequent sea voyage or a rather unpredictable flight by Tanzania Airlines was augmented in 1992 by a catamaran service, operated by a Russian company, which made the journey several times a day. Apart from the convenience of the service to the general public, it brought a more steady stream of tourists to Zanzibar and stimulated the opening of attractive private hotels. At Dar es Salaam the facilities for tourists improved steadily and small charter aircraft could be hired from private companies for flights to almost any part of the country. In other spheres of activity comparable improvements in the quality of life were also being effected by private enterprise.

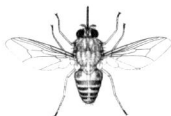

CHAPTER TWENTY-THREE

Looking Back, and Forward

Reflections on the positive and negative impact the relationship with Europe has had on Africa, and Tanganyika specifically - politically, economically and at a humanitarian level. Analysis of the colonial infrastructure, the increase in human population, racial relations, preparation for independence and the colonial withdrawal, early days of independence. A reflection on what the future holds for Africa in view of the widening gap between the developing world and the West. What will be the consequences of economic inequality, growing populations, over-utilised land, civil wars and mass migration?

S ince the day I first stepped off the *T 75* onto African soil in 1944, the continent of Africa has occupied a special place in my heart. Indeed, there have been few years during my career when I have not travelled in one capacity or another to one, or more, African nation. I have witnessed many political changes over those years and have seen at first hand the impact of history upon the people, animals and the land. In recent years I have had the opportunity to reflect upon my observations and experiences and feel I can offer a perspective on what I consider to be some of the merits and demerits of colonial and post-colonial rule in Tanganyika/Tanzania in particular.

In retrospect, the indigenous people of former German East Africa were fortunate that Great Britain was granted a League of Nations Mandate which was formally agreed in July 1922 for the administration of what, at that point, became Tanganyika Territory. Following the end of the First World War there had been an unseemly, latter-day international scramble for the former German territory, practically all of which at that time was occupied by the British forces. The main participants were Belgium, Portugal, the Union of South Africa and, of course, Great Britain. During negotiations between these powers it was proposed that an extensive area of southern Portuguese East Africa should be transferred to the Union of South Africa. In exchange Portugal was to be given the southern half of German East Africa, probably right up to the Central Railway line. Such an arrangement would have imposed the harsh rule of the Portuguese on the indigenous people of the area for the next fifty-five years. They would also have had to endure the many years of gruelling guerrilla warfare that preceded the exodus of the Portuguese in 1975 and the subsequent civil war. Within the above arrangement the northern half of German East Africa would have become a British Colony. Although the indigenous people would have been saved from most of the racism and attendant ill-treatment that they had experienced in German East Africa, there would almost certainly have been further alienation of land for European settlement under British rule and perhaps even amalgamation with Kenya Colony. The League of Nations Mandate saved them from all that.

The Mandate, as quoted by Harlow and Chilver (1965), gave Britain *inter alia* full powers of legislation and administration while binding her to promote to the utmost the material and moral well-being and social progress of the indigenous people, to eliminate domestic and other slavery, to prohibit all forms of forced labour except for public works and services and then only in return for adequate remuneration. In this context, the indigenous people were to be protected against abuse and measures of fraud and force by the careful supervision of labour contracts. No native land was to be transferred, except between indigenous people, without the previous consent of the public authorities. Citizens of all member states of the League were to have the same rights as British citizens in the territory. In order to ensure that the conditions applying to the Mandate were being implemented the British Government was required to report annually to the Council of the League of Nations.

During the run up to the granting of the mandate the British Colonial Office had held the view that the country should be developed primarily for Africans and subsequently favoured the introduction of indirect rule along the general lines of the Nigerian model. Accordingly, in 1925 Sir Donald Cameron, a Caribbean creole of Irish extraction, was transferred from Nigeria to Tanganyika, and in due course he introduced indirect rule. Essentially, indirect rule was a form of local government operated by Native Authorities which, ideally, were headed by a tribal chief supported by a council. Sir Donald saw this as a way of involving the indigenous people in the administration of their own country. The authorities were given legislative and executive powers, native courts and treasuries. The latter were empowered to collect taxes and to retain a proportion of the income for the provision of services and local works; the rest was paid to the central government. For administrative purposes the country was divided into seven Provinces, each of which was headed by a Provincial Commissioner, while the Districts within each Province were in the charge of District Commissioners or District Officers. At this level the District Officers liaised with and supervised the Native Authorities. The Provincial Commissioners reported to the Chief Secretary of the Government, as did the heads of the professional and technical Departments such as Veterinary Science and Animal Husbandry, Agriculture, Medicine, Tsetse Research and Public Works.

Within this arrangement the Department of Veterinary Science and Animal Husbandry worked extremely well, largely because full authority for the administration of the Department was handed down by the Governor through the Chief Secretary to its Director. As I have stated earlier, most Directors as young men had served their apprenticeships in the field, often for long periods under canvas, in close contact with the indigenous people and with the environment in which they and their animals lived. This delegation of authority directly to the Director and through him to his Veterinary Officers and their Livestock Officers encouraged innovation and had a profound effect on the efficiency and the morale of the Department. In view of the paucity of its resources and the formidable problems which it had to tackle in such an immense, underdeveloped country its accomplishments were at the time beyond compare. That situation contrasted markedly with what I subsequently experienced during three years in the Irish Department of Agriculture where the Secretary of the Department was interposed between the Minister and the Director of Veterinary Services. Within this arrangement, which had been inherited from the British, the Secretary and his hierarchy of administrators, devoid of veterinary expertise and even field experience, ran the show whereas the Director was to a large extent an adviser. His staff, apart from those operating the laboratory services, were designated Veterinary Inspectors and, in those days, as the name implied, they merely enforced legislation relating to the control of communicable diseases and meat inspection. There was little incentive or encouragement for the veterinary inspectors to initiate new enterprises. The system was so stultifying that after three years I escaped to Nigeria where, ironically, in due course I saw the same civil service structures being imported from the United Kingdom in preparation for Independence.

The degree of autonomy enjoyed by the Tanganyikan Department of Veterinary Science and Animal Husbandry was, of course, also enjoyed by the other technical Departments. A crude measure of their collective success, and particularly that of the Medical Department, with the meagre resources at their disposal for improving the welfare of the indigenous people, is the increase in the human population that occurred during the first three decades of British rule. Towards the end of German rule in East Africa the population of what was to become Tanganyika was almost certainly less than 4 million. During the military campaign that followed, both sides had plundered so much grain and cattle that by the time the Germans were driven out of German East Africa in 1917 all reserves of food were exhausted. At the end of that year the rains failed and a terrible famine, accompanied by an epidemic of smallpox and flu, held the country in its grip. Despite the appalling number of deaths that occurred at that juncture, the population of Tanganyika had recovered and risen to approximately 5 million by 1931. By 1948 it had reached 7.4 million (Iliffe, 1979); thereafter, it escalated.

The spectacular rise in the human population created its own problems. For example, the periodic failure of the rains followed by famine had always been a feature of the climate especially in Central Tanganyika. This pattern continued at frequent intervals in various parts of the country during the twenties, thirties and forties. Consequently, with increasing numbers of mouths to feed the country was on several occasions on the brink of even more devastating famines accompanied by high mortalities. However, although hardship did occur all too frequently in the more susceptible areas, the type of calamities that had occurred in the past were largely avoided, thanks to the efforts of the technical Departments working through the Provincial Administrations and the Native Authorities. This was achieved in varying degrees by the encouragement given by the

Department of Agriculture to subsistence farmers to grow reserves of drought-resistant manioc and millet. To a lesser extent, the destocking of over-grazed grassland, the provision of grazing reserves cleared of tsetse fly and, later on, the building of reservoirs by the Veterinary Department reduced the morbidity and mortality rates of livestock and consequently the morbidity of man below what they might otherwise have been. But, most of the credit is probably due to the Public Works Department, the District Officers and the Native Authorities for the extensive network of earth roads that was established and subsequently repaired at the beginning of each dry season. Though these roads left much to be desired during normal rainy seasons, relief supplies from other less severely affected areas that were distributed along these roads drastically reduced the incidence of famine. Without them, the distribution of relief food would have been impossible. Consequently, it is fair to say that during the British administration Tanganyika was spared the human misery that is now caused by the devastating famines in sub-Saharan Africa that are currently seen so frequently on our television screens.

Pax Brittanica also ruled supreme; the Wagogo people, who had traditionally lived in fear of Masai cattle raiders, had nothing to fear. In contrast to the situation that developed in post-colonial Tanzania, highway robbery was unheard of and one could travel about after dark with impunity; provided there were no lions or leopards about. Furthermore, at a more extreme level, the appalling genocide that occurred in 1998 in Rwanda would probably never have taken place under colonial rule.

At the personal level the relationship between whites and blacks was, with the inevitable exception of some individuals, free of the racism that was so evident in Northern Rhodesia and Southern Rhodesia. Perhaps the best that one can say about the latter is that it was not as bad as the cruel extremes to which South Africa eventually went in enforcing complete segregation of the races. By comparison, in Tanganyika the relationship between the Masai and European officials was one of mutual respect, tinged perhaps with a slight feeling of superiority on the part of the Masai! At the other end of the scale, the attitude of Europeans to their house servants and indigenous people in general was warmly paternalistic. In retrospect, however, it cannot be denied that some degree of colonialism was evident in the social relationships in the Tanganyika of those days.

For example, it was surely insensitive that mature, often elderly, house servants, who were generally held in affectionate respect by the members of their own families and by the Europeans for whom they worked, were unthinkingly referred to as 'house boys'. To quote a specific case, it also seems to have been quite wrong that Dr Dikshit, the physician and surgeon who served all the Mpwapwa residents – black, white and Asian – so competently and who was always welcome to give as good as he got on the tennis court with the whites, was designated officially as a Sub-Assistant Surgeon just because his medical degree was from an Indian university! Surely, His Majesty's Colonial Service should have had the sensitivity to drop the double negative by omitting, at least, the prefix 'Sub'!

While credit is due to the dedication of so many of the colonial officials who, separated from their families for long periods at a time, devoted their working lives to the development of Tanganyika and the welfare of its people, it should not be overlooked that the British Government's involvement in Tanganyika was not motivated exclusively by altruism. After all, Great Britain was an imperial power with vested interests in retaining overseas territories for purposes such as defence, access to raw materials and other commodities at preferential prices, and the protection of markets for British exports. Consequently, it was expedient to put independence for Tanganyika on the long finger, notwithstanding the fact that it was a Trust Territory. Nevertheless, even if Great Britain had wished to prepare Tanganyika for home rule at a relatively early date and to meet the inevitable cost of doing so it must be recognised that it would have been difficult to refute the argument that charity begins at home. Therefore, it is only fair to recall that while the whole of Europe was recovering from the First World War there was great social deprivation in Great Britain during the twenties as exemplified by mass unemployment of ex-service men and by the coal miners' strike. This was followed by the Great Depression of the thirties which brought about retrenchment of European personnel and the cessation of recruitment in Tanganyika and elsewhere.

One of my memories of the extent to which the Depression and the consequent collapse of world trade affected the U.K. economy was acquired on an occasion when, as a teenager, I travelled with my brother from Dublin to Glasgow during the thirties. As we steamed up the Firth of

Clyde past the Isle of Arran we had a spectacular view of hundreds of redundant, moth-balled merchant ships riding high at anchor in the Sound of Bute and elsewhere; further on, towards Clydebank the silence of the shipyards, from where the bustle and noise of riveting had previously heralded the approach to Glasgow, was awe-inspiring. Equally sobering was a huge abandoned hull, the foetus of the Queen Mary, which was to become the largest luxury liner in the world, with not a worker to be seen. When we disembarked at the Broomielaw, a feature of street scenes was groups of unemployed dockers wearing their traditional peak caps and white mufflers, idling their time away, with the regular 'corner boys' of the time.

In these circumstances it was understandable that the needs of Tanganyika would be neglected. But after the war, even while economic circumstances were still difficult, British taxpayers, in their own interests, had been able to raise £36 million between 1947 and 1950, for the disastrous Groundnut Scheme. Admittedly, during the subsequent seven years approximately £25 million from colonial development funds was allocated to Tanganyika. Perhaps significantly, while most of this was spent on infrastructural development, very little was allocated to education indicating that no serious attention was being given to the preparation of the country for independence. Consequently, according to Iliffe (1979), when Independence came in 1961 there was not even one African Provincial Commissioner, only two of the fifty-seven District Commissioners were Africans. Not one of the thirty-two government veterinarians were Africans. By 1962, only one out of eighty-four civil engineers, two out of fifty-seven lawyers, and sixteen out of 184 physicians were Africans. It would take many years for the ratios to narrow because at that point only forty-five per cent of children were at lower primary schools, nine per cent at upper primary and fewer than two per cent were attending secondary schools. Moreover, it was thought that only sixteen per cent of the population was literate. In retrospect, this abject failure of the British Government to prepare the country for self-government, particularly in the crucial field of education, after no less than thirty-nine years of trust, given initially by the League of Nations and then by the United Nations Organisation, seems to have been, at the least, reprehensible if not inexcusable. The paternalism shown so consistently by Europeans to their servants at a local level should also have been emulated, at the level of governance, by Westminster. The least that middle-aged 'house boys' and their like might have expected was to see their trustees, allocating significantly greater resources for the education of their children. Had more been done in good time to provide a substantial, well-educated middle class, many of the calamities that attended the first twenty-five years of self-government might well have been avoided.

Whatever about the condition the colonial authorities left the country in, the impact of Julius Nyerere's socialism also had a deleterious effect on the autonomous state. I have written in my previous chapter of the advent of Independence in 1961 and what I witnessed of the stranglehold Nyerere's particular strain of socialism had on the young Tanzania. Although the livestock development project on Pemba had done much to improve the welfare of the cooperating smallholders it had done little, if anything, to ease the relentlessly increasing pressure of the human population on the limited arable land available on the island. This, in my opinion, is the fundamental problem threatening the inhabitants of Pemba in the years ahead, just as it is on the mainland of Tanzania and in sub-Saharan Africa generally.

On mainland Tanzania, the human population was approximately four million in 1922 when the British Government was granted the League of Nations Mandate. By 1960, it was estimated to have risen to ten million and in 1997 it reached almost thirty million. At that point it was projected to continue to rise at a rate of 2.56% per annum. One of the consequences of this population explosion, which of course is not confined to Tanzania, has been referred to by the late Kenneth Blaxter (1993), a former Director of the Rowett Research Institute at Aberdeen, Scotland. According to him the population of sub-Saharan Africa has already outrun the present carrying capacity of the land in fourteen countries, which together account for half the population and a third of the land of the whole area of the south of the Sahara. Even with vastly improved technology, seven of these countries cannot reach even a bare self-sufficiency by the year 2000, let alone aspire to the higher nutritional standards which, on the grounds of equity of food provision for all people, can be regarded as necessary. An analysis of possible future trends in world populations, published recently by Lutz Wolfgang *et al.* in the prestigious scientific journal 'Nature' (2001), predicts that despite the prevalence of

HIV in sub-Saharan Africa the population of the area is likely to double during the first fifty years of the present century.

The pressure being exerted on the land by the escalating human population is currently drastically impoverishing, not only the people themselves, but also the fauna and flora of vast areas of the continent and the integrity of the very soil itself on which they depend. These changes are to be seen particularly clearly in the north where the sands of the Sahara are moving several kilometres every year towards the south. As the process continues the surplus population moves from congested land that can no longer sustain them to the shanty towns surrounding the burgeoning cities in search of jobs that do not exist.

However, it is encouraging to find that now, and even before September 11th, some of the world's most powerful international financiers and mega-rich businessmen are, for a variety of reasons, beginning to apply their genius and their influence to the alleviation of problems affecting impoverished sub-Saharan countries. There is growing criticism of the past performance of the United Nations, the World Bank and particularly the International Monetary Fund which, in the case of the latter, is claimed to have been more involved in protecting the interests of the lenders rather than those of their debtors in the Third World. The movement for the elimination of debts involving loans that should never have been granted in the first place by hard-headed bankers, is gaining momentum, as is pressure for the promotion of democracy accompanied by the transfer of capital from the richest countries to the grievously impoverished ones on the periphery of the global economy. Movement away from complete dependence on subsistence farming towards a more diversified economy, which such a transfer of capital would assist, just might raise the standard of living to a level at which human fertility would fall to a more acceptable level as has happened elsewhere in the industrial world. Sadly, if movement in this direction should fail, it will probably remain for the cruel hand of nature to adjust the balance by such natural disasters as devastating famines, AIDS, other diseases as yet unknown and local wars involving boy soldiers with kalashnikovs put into their hands by evil men hungry for power.

The problems of the continent of Africa are being brought home more graphically than before to those of us in the affluent countries of the western world as we encounter the increasing numbers of political refugees and economic migrants among us. The awful plight of those who have fled and those who are left behind is understandably felt more poignantly by individuals who have lived amongst the ordinary people of the stricken African countries. Such individuals, on their return to the frivolities of market-driven affluence at home, recall the endearing qualities of ordinary men and women at the bottom of the pile in Africa; qualities such as their love for their children, their kindness to each other, their affectionate regard for expatriates with whom they have worked or otherwise been in close contact and, above all, their cheerful resilience in the face of awful adversity.

The alleviation, not to mention the solution, of poverty in sub-Saharan Africa and indeed in other areas of the Third World is, of course, so difficult that the present situation may never change, other than for the worse. There are, however, emerging glimmers of hope. While it is generally recognised that the capitalism of the nineties, driven by market forces, has brought great material benefits to the now affluent countries of the world, there is a growing dissatisfaction with the excesses of that system when viewed against the background of the disparity between the haves and the have-nots within our global economy. It does seem quite wrong, and now clearly perilous, that countries which have benefited most from this market-driven global economy are now squandering an inordinate proportion of the world's riches, in the form of sophisticated human skills and material resources, in such a profligate manner when there is so much need for these resources elsewhere. Some of the extent to which such resources are misused can be seen every day in the media as our massive advertising industry strives to promote competing brands of precisely similar products, many of which are patently frivolous. In doing so, it aims to create quite unnecessary new wants while the less profitable basic needs of our global society are largely ignored.

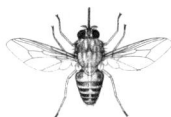

Select Bibliography

Blaxter, Kenneth L., 'Veterinary medicine beyond 2000', in A. R. Michell (ed.), *The Advancement of Veterinary Science,* Bicentenary Symposium Series, (Vol. 1, 1993) pp. 195-205. Reprinted in *Irish Veterinary Journal* **50**, pp. 99-103.

Donnelly, W. J. C., and M. L. Monaghan, *A Veterinary School to Flourish: The Veterinary College of Ireland 1900-2000*, University College Dublin, 2001.

Harlow, Vincent, and E. M. Chilver, assisted by Alison Smith, *History of East Africa*, London, Oxford University Press, 1965.

Iliffe, John, *A Modern History of Tanganyika*, Cambridge University Press, 1979.

Lowe, H. J., 'Rinderpest in Tanganyika', *Empire Journal of Experimental Agriculture* **10** (1942), pp. 189-202.

Newson-Smith, Sue, *Quest: The story of Stanley and Livingstone told in their own words*, London, Arlington Books, 1978.

Stanley, Henry M., *How I Found Livingstone*, London, Sampson Low, Marston, Low, and Searle, 1872.

Lutz, Wolfgang, Warren Sanderson and Sergi Scherlov, 'The End of World Population Growth', *Nature* **412** (2001), pp. 543-545.

Wood, Alan, *The Groundnut Affair, London, The Bodley Head, 1950.*